Get Up and Go

GET | AND
UP | GO

Strategies for Active Living After 50

JIM AND OLGA
McDONALD

THE DUNDURN GROUP
TORONTO · OXFORD

Copy-Editor: Jennifer Bergeron
Design: Jennifer Scott
Printer: University of Toronto Press

National Library of Canada Cataloguing in Publication Data

McDonald, Jim
    Get up and go : strategies for active living after 50 / Jim and Olga McDonald.

ISBN 1-55002-450-7

1. Middle aged persons — Health and hygiene. I. McDonald, Olga II. Title.

RA777.5 M32 2003   613'.0434   C2003-900345-0

1   2   3   4   5   07   06   05   04   03

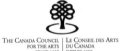   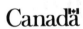

THE CANADA COUNCIL | LE CONSEIL DES ARTS
FOR THE ARTS | DU CANADA
SINCE 1957 | DEPUIS 1957

Canada

ONTARIO ARTS COUNCIL
CONSEIL DES ARTS DE L'ONTARIO

We acknowledge the support of the **Canada Council for the Arts** and the **Ontario Arts Council** for our publishing program. We also acknowledge the financial support of the **Government of Canada** through the **Book Publishing Industry Development Program** and **The Association for the Export of Canadian Books**, and the **Government of Ontario** through the **Ontario Book Publishers Tax Credit** program, and the **Ontario Media Development Corporation's Ontario Book Initiative.**

Care has been taken to trace the ownership of copyright material used in this book. The author and the publisher welcome any information enabling them to rectify any references or credit in subsequent editions.

J. Kirk Howard, President

Printed and bound in Canada.⊛
Printed on recycled paper.
www.dundurn.com

Dundurn Press
8 Market Street
Suite 200
Toronto, Ontario, Canada
M5E 1M6

Dundurn Press
73 Lime Walk
Headington, Oxford,
England
OX3 7AD

Dundurn Press
2250 Military Road
Tonawanda NY
U.S.A. 14150

This book is dedicated to the
Seniors For Nature Canoe Club of Toronto.

From its beginnings in 1984 the club has promoted a full outdoor and social experience that includes canoeing, hiking, cycling, cross-country skiing, and camping. We feel privileged to be members of this vibrant organization. For more information about the club, visit its Web site at www.sfncc.org or send an e-mail to sfncc@rogers.com.

DISCLAIMER

The material presented in this book is for general informational purposes only. The reader should not rely on the information in this book as a substitute for professional medical advice. If you need medical advice you should contact your doctor or another health care professional.

You are personally responsible for any actions you take as a result of using information in this book. If, as a result of reading this book, you participate in a sport or physical activity and sustain an injury or have any other problem, the authors and the publisher will not be held responsible.

CONTENTS

Dreams do come true. I know this because the dream of making the years after 50 the best years of his life came true for my uncle, Jim McDonald. Fifteen years ago, Jim was a smoker with little time for exercise. He was also recovering from open-heart surgery. His doctor advised him to change his lifestyle or risk additional health problems. Jim knew that the advice was sound and he was determined to followed it, one step at a time. He quit smoking, improved his diet, joined a canoe club, and met Olga, his future wife. In the process he discovered that he had to be his own guide. For Jim, this turning point marked the start of the best part of his life.

Get Up and Go is written for older adults who want to change their lives. For some, the motivation may be to improve their health. Others may feel dissatisfied with their sedentary lifestyle. Most people know when they are unhappy with their lives but feel powerless to change the situation. Through honest, personal insights, Jim and Olga guide us through this change. This book encourages people with health problems to adopt a healthier lifestyle, challenges the bystanders of life to stop watching the world pass them by, and helps those planning for retirement to maximize their opportunities.

As a doctor, I found the book's course of action to be inspiring. The book is designed to be interactive. You set your own goals, are praised for your effort, and are encouraged to continue. Here's the exciting news: when you feel better, you look better and become more interesting to be around. Before long you are hooked on life, fuelled by the internal and external rewards of a more active lifestyle. I found that I too was taking stock and thinking of what I could do to improve my lifestyle. While the book is geared for those over 50, the under-50 group can also benefit from this wisdom. It's the kind of guide that allows people of any age to empower themselves.

This book has an important message for those who are retiring: don't just view retirement as the time to put your feet up and relax. Given that retirement can last one-third of your life, making the most of this period is paramount. This book teaches you how to stay active and engaged in life. If you know a relative or friend who is about to retire, this book makes a wonderful retirement gift.

Paula A. Rochon, MD, MPH, FRCPC
Scientist, Kunin Lunenfeld Applied Research Unit,
Baycrest Centre for Geriatric Care

and Associate Professor,
Department of Medicine and Public Health Sciences
University of Toronto

ACKNOWLEDGEMENTS

Since this is an extensive list, I am reassured that most people are kind-hearted and enjoy helping those in need.

First and foremost, a special thanks to Dr. Chris Feindel, whose surgical skills gave me a second chance at life, and a huge thank you to Dr. Paula A. Rochon for so graciously writing the Foreword.

A special thanks to the following:

- Cora L. Craig, president of Canadian Fitness and Lifestyle Research Institute, for reviewing selected parts of the book and providing valuable suggestions;

- Diana Simpson and Rick Hadden, recreation analysts with the City of Mississauga, for reviewing Part One of the book for accuracy; and

- My son, Peter McDonald, of Project Design & Development, Toronto, for his creativity and meticulous care in the development our Web site, www.after50.ca, a fitting promotional enhancement to this book.

Thanks to friends from the Seniors for Nature Canoe Club for their words of wisdom to readers who are searching for a more active lifestyle. I refer to: Cato Bayens, Ethel Corbyn, Ray Crites, Joan Duncan, John Galbraith, Margaret Ghattas, Ken Holden, Renate Juelich, Stewart McTavish, Bea Parkes, and Louise Tye.

The genealogy chapter would be less than complete without quotes taken from thank-you notes received from these family members across Canada and the U.S.: Bettie Alberts, Marjorie Alberts, Ted & Pat Alberts, Valerie Griffith, Bernadine Harper, Nick & Pat Hertz, Grace Jerome, Grace Kennedy, Heather & Louis Kolla, Mary Laski, Adeline Pekar, Rita Pruitt, Margaret & Doug Sleeth, and Pat & Bill Tonita.

A special thanks to the following for their contributions on topics they know so well: Bruce Deachman for Curling, Jean Donato for "A Remarkable Experience," my son Dave McDonald for Cycling, Mary A. Rochon for "Would You Like to be a Docent?", Marlane Tibbs for the "Journey of Learning," and Gerda Tismer for Cross-Country Skiing.

"All we need to make us happy is something to be enthusiastic about."
— Charles Kingsley (1819–1875), British writer

Knock, Knock
Who's there?
Nobody!

No one is going to come knocking at your door or send you an invitation to join a venture guaranteed to improve your health and your outlook on life. It's not going to happen, so don't wait. You have to take the initiative; you have to make it happen. If you are waiting for a more opportune time to start doing something about your inactivity, don't wait for that, either, because there will never be a perfect time — the best time is now. As someone once said, "It may not be your fault that you are down, but it's your duty to get up."

You have taken the first step by picking up this book, so flip through the pages, get acquainted with it, start reading, and allow the book to lead you toward a longer, more enjoyable life. You won't find any quick fixes in this book. Nor will you find any discussion of herbs, diets, or natural supplements. But you will find out how to keep your body fit and your mind active. Our aim is a healthier, happier life for everyone after fifty.

Early on in the book you will learn that more than half of Canadian adults are inactive. That is, they do not exercise enough to benefit their health. That's a scary statistic, for that kind of idleness is killing us. But there's more; in the age group 45 to 64, 41 percent of the men and 32 percent of the women are overweight. And among these overweight people, 16 percent are obese!

In 1998 Health Canada launched its "Physical Activity Guide" for the general population and another issue for "older adults" a year later. The purpose of the guides was to encourage Canadian adults to become more active. In addition, all levels of government responsible for fitness, recreation, and sport set a goal to decrease by 10 percent the number of inactive Canadians by 2003. Slowly, they are making headway.

Our Goal: Help Make It Happen

Our main purpose in writing this book is to motivate the 50-plus group to become more physically and mentally active, thus contributing to Health Canada's 10 percent goal.

In the year 2002:

- 9 million Canadians (29 percent) were over the age of 50
- 4 million Canadians (12.6 percent) were over the age of 65

Statistics Canada advises that by 2026 the over-65 group will increase to 21 percent of the population, giving us 8 million Canadians over age 65. This rapid increase in the seniors population is attributed to increased life expectancy and the entry of baby boomers into the seniors age group.

Here's a statistic that will take some getting used to: The number of working-age people per senior has been falling for some time. In 2000 there were eight working-age persons for each senior; by 2026 there will be just five working-age persons for each senior. Imagine a population with a "support ratio" of five working people to one senior.

The High Cost of Inactivity

From the abundance of proof that inactivity increases health care costs, here is just one statement to make the point.

"Hot Topics in Physical Activity," a report produced by Health Canada's SummerActive campaign, quotes the following, which is part of a larger report, "Effective Active Living Interventions" (John C. Spence, 2001), submitted to Health Canada on behalf of the Canadian Consortium of Health Promotion Research. You can find the report on-line at www.gov.ab.ca/acn/200206/12646.html.

Physical inactivity is associated with chronic diseases (e.g., colon cancer, diabetes, cardiovascular disease) that are part of the economic burden on the health-care system. Physically active adults are more likely to experience a higher quality of life and less functional decline in old age than inactive adults, reducing the burden on the health-care system.

In 1999, the direct health-care costs in Canada of physical inactivity totaled $2.1 billion. These costs of physical inactivity represented approximately 25 percent of the health-care costs of diseases linked to physical inactivity.

The Resting Mode

We all strive for periods of comfort and relaxation. And once retirement arrives, some people visualize and indeed pursue a lifetime of leisure with their minds and bodies at rest. They do nothing, and they become content in their resting mode, resisting any kind of activity. In the meantime their bodies and minds deteriorate from lack of use. Today, 62 percent of our seniors are in this mode.

They have forgotten how much more invigorating and satisfying life can be when their body moves and their mind is at work.

It is imperative that we find a way to dislodge these men and women from the sedentary lifestyle they have grown accustomed to. Health Canada's "Physical Activity Guide" for seniors is a good beginning, but there has to be more. Most provincial governments produce booklets with titles such as "Seniors' Guide to Services and Programs." These booklets place heavy emphasis on health, drugs, ambulance, foot care, old age security benefits, and hearing aids, but say precious little about how to keep a healthy body and an active mind. One province packed everything it had to say about active living into thirteen lines of its booklet.

How to Use This Book

We suggest that you read the first part of this book in sequence from Chapter 1 to Chapter 4. That way you will encounter Chapter 2: Take Charge of Your Life and Chapter 4: Set Your Goals early on. Read the rest of the book in any sequence you wish. As you read this book you may wish to keep a highlighter handy so you can mark the areas of special interest for quick reference later on.

Information about caring for your mind and body goes far beyond the confines of this book. Thus, here and there throughout the book we have included Web site addresses (URLs) that will allow you to explore a host of topics in greater detail at your own convenience. Inevitably, some URLs will no longer work. We must expect that, for Web sites addresses are often changed, and sometimes Web sites are closed down altogether.

Part One: Active Body establishes our primary motivation for writing this book: the shockingly high rate of inactivity among Canadian adults. This part of the book also provides for a self-assessment of your own level of physical activity and shows you how to set your own lifetime goals and establish an activity program that meets your needs.

As you proceed through the book we hope you will get involved by completing several worksheet activities designed to start you actively thinking about an improved lifestyle. We also provide dozens of examples of activities to choose from and several detailed descriptions of specific sports, written by enthusiasts who love what they do.

Part Two: Active Mind discusses the need to keep your mind active and healthy. In this second part, our purpose is to provide an in-depth look at several broad areas of involvement that have brought mental stimulation and fulfillment to thousands of over-50 men and women in recent years. Again we include activities here and there to help you identify your own areas of interest. Throughout this second part we examine volunteering, computers, genealogy, adult education, and arts, crafts, and hobbies.

Visit Our Web Site

As you read through this book you will find references to more than 100 Web sites. Normally, the only way to open these sites would be to manually key in each URL. But here's a better way: go to our Web site, www.after50.ca, and you will find a categorized list of all the Web sites mentioned in this book. Then, simply click on the Web site of your choice. When it opens, you can save it to your own list of favourites. At our Web site you will also find links to more sites you'll be interested in, an area for ordering books, and much more. We'll keep the Web site current and interesting so that you will have reason to visit it again and again.

What We Hope to Accomplish

- Get this message out to everyone over 50: *There's a world of fitness and pleasure out there. All you have to do is go get it.*
- Motivate people 50-plus to:
    - become more physically and mentally active,
    - make active living a way of life,
    - join outdoor clubs, seniors' centres, and fitness centres, and
    - participate in Senior Games in their home province.
- Let Canadians know that most seniors do not have one foot in the grave.
- Spread the message that major surgery may be the beginning of something better, not the end.
- Encourage all employers to make *Get Up and Go* a parting gift to their employees when they retire. They need it!

Sidebars

Throughout the book you will find two types of boxes or sidebars intended to draw your attention to a special quote or comment. Here are the two types.

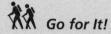 *Go for It!*

Sidebars headed *Go for It!* contain entries from members of the Seniors for Nature Canoe Club. When we first began this book, we considered asking "experts" for quotes on how to keep physically fit and mentally active. Then it occurred to us that the most qualified experts on these topics were the ordinary "active" 55-plus folks within our own canoe club.

We asked some of the members to provide a few words of wisdom for people who are aspiring to become more active. Throughout the book you'll see what they had to say in these sidebars.

 Feedback

These sidebars appear only in Chapter 8: Tracing Your Ancestors. They contain excerpts from letters I received from relatives after they received their copy of the Griffith family history, which I recently completed. The purpose of these sidebars is to show that family history research does have its rewards.

PART ONE: ACTIVE BODY

I'm a lucky guy and I want to pass on some of that good fortune to you. You'll soon see that I have what some describe as a cardiac problem. I prefer to think of it as a stroke of luck. You see, if it hadn't been for my so-called problem I wouldn't be feeling as fit as I do, I wouldn't be associating with so many active people, and Olga and I would not have written this book.

Somebody once said, "If exercise were a pill, it would be the most widely prescribed medicine in the world." Great idea, but we're not there yet. In the meantime, if you want to enjoy your second half you'll have to keep your body moving or it will stop working. As my doctor used to say, "Use it or lose it."

We begin this book by pointing out the sorry state of inactivity we are in, then we ask you to take stock of your own situation. We show you how to take charge of your life, and we get you involved in doing it. You review and select activities of your choice, you set goals for yourself, and you aim for a more fulfilling and active lifestyle. You'll find this book fast-moving, informative, and fun. It may even save your life.

In this chapter:

- Decide what's most important in your life.

- Learn how to gain important health benefits by being active.

- Find out how much exercise is enough — it's less than you think.

- Take stock of your own situation.

If I had known I was going to live this long, I would have taken better care of myself.

> — Eubie Blake, (1883–1983), U.S. songwriter and pianist

Stay Alive and Well

In July 1988 I sat across the desk from Dr. Chris Feindel at the Toronto Western Hospital and listened intently as he explained my upcoming open-heart surgery.

When he said, "Jim, here's what you have to do to stay healthy after surgery," I borrowed a sheet of paper from him to make a few notes of what he was about to say. This was undoubtedly the most important meeting of my life, and I wanted to remember every detail of his instructions.

Although Dr. Feindel is a soft-spoken man, his message came across loud and clear. As a cardiovascular surgeon he was about to save my life — this time — but after surgery, it was my responsibility to do what was necessary to stay alive and well.

When I recently looked at my notes from that meeting I was surprised at the sheer simplicity and brevity of what I wrote down. Here it is, only a few simple words with a powerful message:

1. Don't smoke
2. Eat right
3. Exercise

Since Dr. Feindel was talking about my life, I expected to find more, but that was it! That was the extent of my notes. If heeded, the doctor's three warnings encompassed all that was necessary to promote a healthy lifestyle. Furthermore, his words of wisdom are as valid today as they were back in 1988.

The surgery went well, and like thousands of other bypass patients I was up and around in no time. But I was still faced with the three major challenges: don't smoke, eat right, and exercise. I was at my "fork in the road." Would I make the right choices?

Your Fork in the Road

It sounds simple enough; all I had to do was quit smoking, start eating right, and exercise, but talking about it and doing it are two entirely different kettles of fish. I knew that I had to get those three monkeys off my back or I would just be marking time, waiting to die for the remainder of a very dull life.

You may be in a similar position at age 50 or 80 or somewhere in between. You may be retired or about to retire when out of the blue something happens to make your life less beautiful than it was a few days before. Maybe it was a little thing, like having to move your belt out one more notch to accommodate your increasing girth, or maybe it was a TV commercial or a magazine article that made you acutely aware that you were totally out of shape. Or, God forbid, you had to walk up a flight of stairs and found yourself totally exhausted.

Whatever your situation, you may be at your fork in the road with your own monkeys to shake off. Whether you get a gentle warning about your health, or like me, get hit with a sledge hammer, it's essential that you do something about it, and this book is designed to help you. You have made an excellent start. Stay with us and we'll help you every step of the way toward a healthier, more active lifestyle.

What's Important in Your Life?

Ask anyone over the age of 50, "What's the most important thing in your life?" and I'll wager that most will respond with an unqualified, "My health!" The reason is simple: they want to live longer and enjoy life at the same time.

By the time you hit 50 you know damn well you have more years behind you than you have in front of you, so start paying attention to your health; it's more critical now than ever before.

Wish #1 — Good Health

You instinctively know that unless you're in good health, your joy of living will be greatly diminished. Some people simply trust to luck and hope for the best, while others take steps that will lead to prolonged health. In this chapter we'll show you how to tip the scales of good health in your favour.

Wish #2 — A Longer Life

A while back one of my adult sons said to me, "Well Dad, I guess you should have at least another ten years left." He quickly realized that his comment startled me, so he added, "Or maybe you'll be like your father and live to be one hundred and two." That felt much better. You will have an opportunity to give serious thought to your own life expectancy when you take part in the Longevity Game in Chapter 2.

Stop right now, give some serious thought to the question below, then enter your response. You may want to revisit this page later to see what you entered.

What is most important in your life?

Jot it down here: _____

My Three Monkeys

I don't want to leave you in suspense wondering what happened to my three monkeys, so I'm pleased to let you know that I conquered them all one by one.

Don't Smoke: I kicked the smoking habit soon after I learned of my heart problem. You can't imagine the relief of being freed from that monkey. It was not easy for me to quit, and if you happen to be a smoker it probably won't be easy for you, either. Plan on repeated attempts before you finally win that battle, but keep at it until you have succeeded because it's worth the struggle. That's all I'll say about smoking, because it is not the focus of this book.

Eat Right: Thanks to my wife, Olga, I now "eat right" all the time. Eating right is critical to good health but again it is not the focus of this book. I suggest that you obtain a copy of Health Canada's "Food Guide." It contains guidelines for healthy eating, tips on how to reduce fat, the kinds of foods to choose for healthy eating, how much you need to eat from each food group each day, and much more. To order, contact Health and Welfare Canada, Ottawa, ON, K1A 0K9 or phone 613-954-5995.

Exercise: Dr. Feindel's third admonition to exercise is the focus of this part of the book. Exercise, Exercise, Exercise! You may well ask, "Why all the fuss about exercise?" Here's why: Exercise is the secret to a healthier, happier life in your second half.

The Problem Is Inactivity

In October 2002 the Canadian Fitness and Lifestyle Research Institute (CFLRI), Canada's watchdog for physical activity levels, released a report on the results of the 1998/99 Canadian National Population Health Survey. The report states that:

- 55 percent of adult Canadians are not active enough to benefit their health.

While that's an improvement over previous activity levels, it's still an alarming statistic. It means that more than half of us are couch potatoes. Imagine, more than half of our population is either glued to the television, the computer, or the couch!

The Older Crowd Is Even More Inactive

The CFLRI reports that:

- In the 65-plus age group, 62 percent are physically inactive.

That's a disturbing statistic for an age group whose quality of life is so closely linked to maintaining an active lifestyle.

The Writing Is on the Wall

Not too many years ago most Canadians lived on farms where everyone in the family worked from dawn till dusk just to get through the normal process of living. Today, with our innumerable labour-saving devices, we can easily get through the day without lifting a finger, so to speak. For most people, daily living is totally devoid of any type of exercise or physical activity. We even push a button to open and close the garage door. With the advent of remote control we don't even have to get off our butts to switch TV channels.

On March 17, 2001, the *Toronto Star* headline read:

> We're living the easy life and it's killing us. Increasingly idle, we're becoming increasingly big — and less healthy.

In March 1999, the CFLRI stated that technological advancements have led to increasingly sedentary lifestyles in Canada, with the result that physical inactivity is now a major public health issue. It says, "Our daily lives abound with passive activities at work, and at home."

In 1999, Dr. Francine Lemire, president of the College of Family Physicians of Canada, stated, "If you are inactive, studies show that the health risk could be on par with smoking..." Let's repeat that thought: *Inactivity is as harmful to your health as smoking!*

If you happen to be among the 55 percent of inactive Canadians and you choose to remain inactive:

- Your bone strength will decline,
- Your muscles will get weak and flabby,
- You will lose flexibility in your joints, tendons, and ligaments,
- The efficiency of your heart and lungs will decline, and
- You will be twice as likely to develop coronary heart disease as active people.

Die from Doing Nothing?

Not too long ago, while attending a social event, Olga fell into conversation with a former acquaintance we'll call Charlie. When Olga told me the story of her unusual discussion with Charlie, I knew that I had to include it in this book, for it conveys an attitude that may be secretly shared by others.

When Charlie mentioned that he was now retired, Olga asked him what he was doing with all his spare time. Charlie proudly responded by saying, "I do nothing. I sleep until ten in morning. Once I have breakfast, shower, shave, get dressed, and do a few things, it's time for lunch." He sipped his wine and continued on, "After lunch I go to the club and play cards with guys for the rest of the afternoon. In the evening I watch television." Olga listened in shocked silence as he supported his "do nothing" position with his next statement.

> "Like I said, I do nothing and there's nothing wrong with that. When you read the paper, do you ever see a headline that says someone died from doing nothing? Of course not, nobody dies from doing nothing!"

What an intriguing revelation. Most people who make up the more than half of our inactive population offer excuses for their inactivity and make promises to change their ways in the near future. Not Charlie. He spoke of his "do nothing" lifestyle with the confidence of someone who had just found the secret to longevity. I suspect that Charlie and his buddies at the club share similar views, and they may be typical of many more who live a sedentary lifestyle.

Unfortunately, when Charlie's friends read his obituary, the official cause of his demise will not be described as "doing nothing." His cause of death will indeed be identified as something much more complex, and most will never make the connection to his sedentary lifestyle. In 2002 the World Health Organization said this about those who live Charlie's lifestyle:

> Sedentary lifestyles increase all causes of mortality, double the risk of cardiovascular diseases, diabetes, and obesity and substantially increase the risks of colon cancer, high blood pressure, osteoporosis, depression, and anxiety.

The Benefits of Being Active

Here's what the Canadian Fitness and Lifestyle Research Institute says about the benefits of being active:

- Even a low-to-moderate level of regular activity will decrease the risk of coronary heart disease;
- Physical activity reduces the risk of colon cancer and possibly the risk of breast cancer and lung cancer;
- Physical activity reduces the risk of back problems;
- Physical activity reduces the risk of osteoporosis. Active people have a greater bone mass than inactive people;
- Physical activity reduces the risk of obesity;
- Physical activity reduces anxiety and stress;
- Physical activity helps reduce mild-to-moderate depression;

- Active people tend to be more satisfied with their physical appearance and weight; and
- Regular physical activity that includes interaction with other people is likely to increase enjoyment of life.

Health Canada Takes Up the Challenge

On October 21, 1998, Health Canada and the Canadian Society for Exercise Physiology (SCEP) launched "Canada's Physical Activity Guide to Healthy Active Living." This 27-page handbook provides Canadians with clear and concise guidelines on how to achieve better health by making physical activity an important part of daily living. The guide has been endorsed by 44 national organizations representing health care professionals, parents, educators, recreation organizations, city and town planners, and provincial, territorial, and municipal governments.

> Furthermore, all levels of the government responsible for fitness, recreation, and sport set a goal to decrease by 10 percent the number of inactive Canadians by the year 2003.

At the time of the launching, Mr. Doug MacQuarrie of the Heart and Stroke Foundation of Canada said:

> If Canadians want to keep their hearts healthy as they age and be active in their retirement years, they need to make physical activity as routine as brushing their teeth or putting on their seat belts.

Health Canada Targets Older Adults

In May 1999, "Canada's Physical Activity Guide and Handbook for Older Adults" was launched. It was a new tool, they said, to help stall the effects of aging. And this:

Older adults who maintain an active lifestyle will enjoy better physical and mental health, better posture and balance, more energy, regular sleep patterns, and prolonged living in later years.

Dr. Ira Jacobs, president of the Canadian Society of Exercise Physiology, had this to say:

> We know that up to half of the functional decline that occurs in humans between the age of 30 and 70 is attributable to a sedentary lifestyle, and not aging in itself. ... If used as directed, this new guide, specifically designed for older adults, is as close as we can get to having an anti-aging medication.

A copy of both physical activity guides can be obtained by calling Health Canada's toll free line: 1-888-334-9769, or by visiting: www.paguide.com.

We're Getting Heavier

In 1996, Statistics Canada conducted a national population health survey of over 80,000 adult Canadians. You will be interested in the results of this survey, which reveal more startling statistics about our weight problem.

The following excerpts are from the Canadian Fitness and Lifestyle Research Institute. Please note the significant increase in weight levels from the 25 to 44 age group to the 45 to 64 age group.

> Weight categories are calculated by using the Body Mass Index (BMI). The BMI divides a person's weight in kilograms by height in metres squared.
>
> - Overweight is defined as a BMI greater than 27.
> - Obesity is defined as a BMI greater than 30.

Age Group	Overweight BMI > 27	Obese BMI > 30
Total 25–44	**27**	**11**
Women	29	9
Men	33	13
Total 45–64	**37**	**16**
Women	32	15
Men	41	16

Why We're Getting Bigger

- Probably the most important reason is a decline in daily physical activity. As people age, they tend to be less active than they were in their youth. Technologies such as computers, cable television, cellphones, and VCRs mean that we use less energy in our day-to-day lives.
- Today, our expenditure of physical energy is so small that the food we take in is far in excess of the energy going out. And all that excess goes to fat.
- Our eating patterns have changed. Canadians are much more likely to eat high-calorie fast foods now than we were fifteen years ago. Fast food chains are everywhere.
- Gaining weight as you age is common but not inevitable. Many people who stay active and eat a healthy, moderate diet manage to maintain the weight of their youth into their 40s, 50s, and 60s.

The Magic Level of Physical Activity

Health Canada states that you should be active enough to benefit your health. But how active is that? Exactly how much physical activity is necessary to achieve the desired health benefits? How much energy do we have to expend? Since every person's situation is different, we can't say exactly how much exercise is right for you. But thanks to scientific research and Health Canada's physical activity guides, we do have some general guidelines. As a minimum, here is what Health Canada recommends for both "adults" and "older adults":

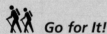 **Go for It!**

Active people live longer, stay healthier, and enjoy a better quality of life. I also think they are more interesting.
— Louise Tye

Engage in 30 minutes of moderate activity at least 4 days a week. The 30 minutes can be accumulated in 10 minute segments.

Always consult with your doctor or health care professional before beginning an exercise program.

I think you will agree that these recommendations do not appear threatening. A minimum of 30 minutes a day, 4 days a week sounds easy enough. That's only a brisk 30-minute walk, 30 minutes of invigorating swimming, or 30 minutes of active housework! And that 30 minutes does not have to be done all at once: three 10-minute segments of activity at different times during the day count for 30 minutes of activity.

But more than half of us don't even do that much for our health. A leisurely 15-minute walk to the store twice a week won't cut it, because you are not expending enough energy to benefit your body. Health Canada's guidelines tell us how much physical activity is necessary to benefit our health, eliminating the speculation about how much exercise is "enough." We can strive to meet these guidelines and adapt them to our own unique situation. You now know that you have to do more than a 15-minute leisurely walk to the store, but you also know you don't have to sign up for daily 2-hour workouts at the gym.

You now know that you can turn that leisurely walk into an activity that will benefit your health. Gradually pick up the pace, increase the distance and the frequency until your former stroll becomes a 30-minute brisk walk 4 times a week. The key word here is "gradual." Don't push yourself too hard when you begin a change in your level of activity. Take it easy so that both your body and your mind can adjust. By easing into your increased activity you are more likely to stick with it over the long haul.

Return on Investment

Looking at it from a different perspective, if you exercise for 30 minutes, 4 days a week you get back 168 hours of healthy living for an investment of only 2 hours. Do your own math to check it out. Just keep making those weekly two-hour deposits and your body will respond with seven days of enjoyable living week after week. No matter what your age or how long you have been inactive, exercise will always improve your physical condition. Do it, and in no time at all you will feel the improvement.

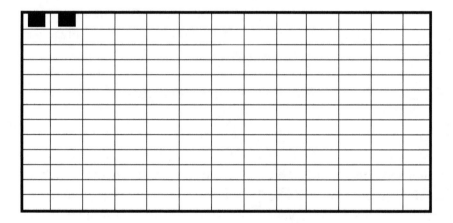

The squares above represent the 168 hours in a week. If you build moderate activity into your daily routine for a minimum of 30 minutes, 4 days a week (that's 2 hours a week) as indicated in the top left-hand corner of the chart, it will improve your health and fitness. Just 2 hours of input and you're covered for 168. What a bargain!

Why Are We So Inactive?

So why aren't people more active? Why don't we exercise when we know it's necessary for good health? In the past few years we have been inundated with information related to health and healthy living by every form of media, including newspapers, radio, television, booklets, and the Internet. By now, we should be well aware of our body's need for exercise, but most of us still fail to respond.

Maybe the 50-plus group will react if the message is presented in a different format. That's what we hope to accomplish with this book.

According to the 1996 national population health survey, more than half (55 percent) of Canadians stated they should do something about their health. That is, they felt they should become more physically active, quit smoking, lose weight, or improve their eating habits.

Almost half of those who stated they should be doing more physical activity to improve their health also said there was something stopping them from becoming more physically active. Here are some of the reasons reported in that survey. Check off the barriers that apply to you so that you can deal with them later on.

 Go for It!

Your mind and attitude should say to you, if it can be done, I can do it. Force your mind to drive your body and make it become active.
— John Galbraith

Excuses, Excuses

Lack of time:
Since this book is aimed at the over-50 segment of the population, lack of time should not be as significant a barrier as it used to be. If you are retired or only work part time, but still cling to "lack of time" as a reason for not being more physically active, you should rethink your priorities. Maybe your lifestyle is out of balance. When you retired, you suddenly found seven or eight hours of additional time every day. Surely you can find 30 minutes, 4 days a week for your body.

Get out a pencil and paper and make a list of what you do during the day and how much time you spend on each major activity. I'll bet you can find 30 minutes each day for your health.

Lack of willpower or self-discipline:

If you know you should be more active for reasons of your health but you can't find the energy to do anything about it, keep reading and you will find plenty of suggestions that will help you get started, as well as tips on how to stay motivated. Maybe the importance of physical activity hasn't sunk in yet, but it will. Focus on the fact that exercise or physical activity will add to your vitality and the quality of your life.

Disability or health problems:

Certainly some Canadians are limited in the amount of exercise they can do because of a physical condition or health problem. If you have a health problem, ask your doctor what would be safe for you. There are a variety of exercise programs available for adults with special needs. Hospitals and various types of community centres conduct special programs for those with heart-related problems, osteoporosis, multiple sclerosis, Parkinson's disease, and more.

Fatigue:

If you are tired of being tired, exercise may be exactly what you need. Start small with a 5- to 10-minute walk and gradually increase your time each day. Do it again tomorrow and again the next day, and before you know it you will be feeling so much better that your outings will not only be enjoyable, they will become part of your daily routine. Here are a few tips:

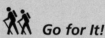 **Go for It!**

Start gradually. Remember, our bodies were not made for rest; they are superbly designed for motion. Once you are over the initial inertia and in the habit of exercise, your body wants to play and is happy when you move it. It will reward you with a feeling of total well-being.

— Margaret Ghattas

- Go to bed a reasonable hour and get the sleep you need.
- Be up and about at a reasonable hour every morning ready to enjoy the new day.
- Do your walking (or other exercise) at a time of the day best suited for you. Many people like to do their activities first thing in the morning before they get involved with something else.

- Find a buddy to join you in your exercise activity. You can give each other support.
- Make it a fun thing. Don't think of your activity as a chore; make it an enjoyable period of your day.

Financial considerations:

If you are serious about becoming more active there are numerous ways to do it without spending a dime. Keep on reading and you'll find that the highest ranking activity — walking — is free.

If over the years you have planned for your retirement by building up a pension and putting aside a few dollars to help you enjoy your later years, you have an obligation to yourself to keep active once you approach that period in your life. If you don't, you are sabotaging your own retirement plans. Why bother with financial retirement plans if you don't have plans for a healthy body?

More Perceived Barriers

Here is another list of reasons often given for not exercising. If you see an item that applies to you, check it off. By the end of the next chapter these barriers should no longer deter you from getting started on the road to activity and health, because you will have learned how to eliminate them.

- Fear of the strange, unknown world of exercise
- Don't know how to get started or who to contact
- Don't have the confidence to start something new
- Fear that physical activity may result in injury or pain
- Don't have a partner
- A feeling that physical activity won't do you any good
- Unaware of how good you will feel after a workout
- Don't have transportation
- You think you won't like it

The Best Time of Your Life

If you maintain your health, your second half can be the best time of your life. Your children have grown up and left the nest and you are now free to do all those wonderful things you never had time to do before. But there is always that nagging concern about health. Of what value is a long life or an abundance of money if health problems remove you from the pursuit of an enjoyable life, especially if your health problems were brought about by inactivity, something you have total control over?

If you're beginning to feel comfortable with a sedentary lifestyle, totally devoid of physical activity, huffing and puffing at every turn, ask yourself, "How long has it been since I felt really great?" It could be that you have forgotten what if feels like to have a zest for life, to be full of energy and bursting with enthusiasm. If so, don't blame your fatigue on age, even if you've hit 60, 70, or more. Old and tired has more to do with attitude, outlook, and lifestyle than the calendar.

Nine million Canadians have passed the 50 year mark. And 45 percent of them are living an active lifestyle. Aim to become a part of that group. We are fortunate to live in a country where a health plan covers the cost of most doctor bills. But your doctor cannot prescribe a magic pill as an exercise replacement — that's your responsibility. If you expect your second half to be the best part of your life, make a commitment to treat yourself to more activity.

Check the Internet

There are hundreds of Web sites that provide excellent information about exercise and fitness as well as other medical information. Here are two sites you may wish to explore:

- Health Canada's site: http://www.hc-sc.gc.ca
- The National Library of Medicine in the U.S.: http://www.medlineplus.gov, a first-rate site that includes information on exercise and fitness

ACTIVITY # 1: TAKING STOCK

As you proceed through this book, there will be several occasions when we ask you to stop for a moment and reflect upon your personal situation. We want you to do that now. Your answers to these questions will tell you whether it's your wake-up time. If so, the remainder of this book will help put direction into your life. Check off your responses.

1. When you first open your eyes in the morning, do you usually view the new day with a feeling of enthusiasm and pleasure?

    yes ____ no ____ sometimes ____

2. At this time, are you involved in a project or pursuing a goal in life?

    yes ____ no ____

3. Are you doing what you can to live a full and meaningful life right now instead of waiting until some time in the future when it feels right?

    yes ____ no ____

4. In the past seven days, how much time have you spent doing some kind of moderate physical activity such as swimming, brisk walking, active housework, cycling, etc.?

    None ____ 30 minutes ____ 1 hour ____ 2 hours ____ Other ____

There are no right or wrong answers. "Yes" responses suggest that you have a sense of direction and a clear purpose in life. "No" responses suggest that you may be on a downhill slide, accepting whatever happens without any intervention on your part. You may be unnecessarily wasting your life, when in fact you have the power to make it more enjoyable.

QUICK SUMMARY

- More than half of the adult Canadian population are physically inactive, and that's a major health issue for both you and the country.

- Health Canada published two booklets, "Canada's Physical Activity Guide to Healthy Active Living" and "Guide for Older Adults," to encourage Canadians to begin a more active lifestyle. Get a copy at a seniors' centre near you.

- At the very least, you should be doing 30 minutes of moderate activity 4 days a week. If you don't, you run the risk of spending the second half of your life in sick bay.

- Most barriers to physical activity can be overcome with a bit of effort, and this book shows you how.

In this chapter:

- Where are you now and where are you headed?

- Draw your own timeline and ponder your future.

- Find out if you are FIT enough to enjoy your future.

- Make your health commitment.

It is not the number of years in your life that is important ... it is the life you put into those years that counts.

— E. Bourque

You Are the Centre of Attention

In the previous chapter, It's Wake-Up Time, we concentrated on the deplorable level of fitness among Canadian adults. In this chapter we shift our emphasis away from the whole nation to you as an individual. We will ask you to focus on yourself and what you are doing to look after your health. Elie Wiesel's poem makes the point.

Where Do I Start?
By Elie Wiesel

But where do I start?
The world is so vast,
I shall start with the country
I know best, my own.
But my country is so large.

I had better start with my town.
But my town, too, is large.
I had best start with my street.
No: my home. No: my family,
Never mind, I shall start with myself.

Yes, we will focus on "you" and we'll try to reach you in such a way that you internalize our activity message and actually want to get up and go. Let's not lose sight of where this book is headed. We want you to enjoy a better, more fulfilling life, and that calls for you to be physically and mentally active. In case you have any doubts about that, let me introduce you to ALCOA and what they have to say.

The Partnership

ALCOA (Active Living Coalition for Older Adults) is a partnership of 26 organizations having an interest in the field of aging and active living in Canada. Their mission is in part "… to encourage older Canadians to maintain and enhance their well-being and independence through a lifestyle that embraces daily physical activities." Just to give you a sampling, 4 of the 26 organizations that partner with ALCOA are: the Canadian Red Cross Society, the College of Family Physicians of Canada, the YMCA, and the Osteoporosis Society of Canada.

In its booklet "A Blueprint for Action," ALCOA sets out nine guiding principles that represent the values, beliefs, and philosophical underpinnings that they hold to be true with respect to an active way of life. We want you to be aware of ALCOA's first guiding principle, for it is also the basic premise of Part One of this book.

ALCOA's First Guiding Principle is:
It is recognized that active living is essential for daily living and a cornerstone of health and quality of life.

Where Are You Now?

Let's diverge for a few moments while we visualize an imaginary trip that has taken you to beautiful Prince Edward Island.

Whenever we take a road trip I always enjoy stopping at the tourist information centres. I'm fascinated by all the brochures, flyers, and maps on display at these places. Most of all I am attracted to the huge map usually affixed to the wall under a covering of glass. Visitors always gravitate to the big map on the wall to find out where they are. Of course, the people in charge of information centres anticipate the travellers' need to know that, so they insert a large "You Are Here" sign on the map with an arrow pointing to wherever you are at that time.

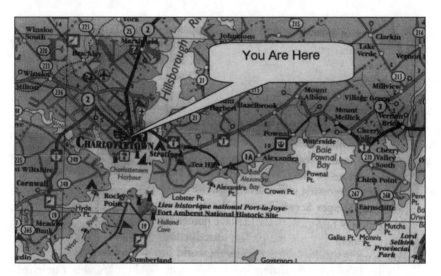

Let's assume you left Brandon, Manitoba four days ago to visit relatives in Tignish, P.E.I. It's been a long but enjoyable drive and you have just arrived in Charlottetown. You want to get more information about P.E.I. so you stop at the Charlottetown Information Centre.

You enter the tourist office and saunter over to the large map on the wall. You see the word Charlottetown at the end of the "You Are Here" arrow, but of course you already knew that because you saw the big Charlottetown sign as you drove into town. The value of the map and the "You Are Here" mark is that it provides you with a point of reference. Knowing where you are on the map allows you to determine where you are in relation to other points of interest. For instance, you can now easily calculate that you must drive another 153 kilometres to reach Tignish.

And so it is in life. This is the most opportune time for you to examine your own map of life from wherever you are at this time. You can look back at where you have been and forward to where you are headed right now and as you proceed through this chapter. If you don't do it now while reading this chapter, you may not get back to it later. We'll guide you each step of the way. The purpose is to help you plan for a well-balanced life that you can live to the fullest.

You Are Here

If you are about to retire in the near future, chances are that you will be hit with a few surprises in the months ahead. You see, retirement is new ground for you, so it's only natural that you are unprepared for what lies ahead. Your working years were different; you

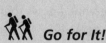 **Go for It!**

Hire a student and pay him or her to walk with you three times a week. You pay the student whether you show up for the walk or not!
— Stewart McTavish

were trained to do the job. If you were unsure of what to do, there were people to call on for help. That's not the way it is in retirement.

If you are already retired you may have been fortunate enough to attend a brief seminar devoted to an "Introduction to Retirement," but that only skimmed the surface of what lay ahead. You probably stumbled into retirement with no particular goals in mind for your new lifestyle. You rejoiced in the realization that you didn't have to get up for work in morning, had no deadlines to meet, no one to report to, and no meetings to prepare for. Retirement was your reward. It was payback time. You put your feet up and relaxed. Life was beautiful.

But gradually your new life begins to lose its charm. Maybe you miss the daily contact with your friends at work. Maybe you miss the challenge, the sense of accomplishment and status that came with your job. Ask yourself:

- Are you bored with life?   Yes ____ No ____
- Is each new day just another yesterday?   Yes ____ No ____
- Do you feel unhappy much of the time?   Yes ____ No ____
- Do you lack the energy to do anything?   Yes ____ No ____

If you answered "yes" to any of these questions it's time to re-examine your life and your priorities. If you are not putting out any energy, there are no rewards flowing back. If you feel lazy, discarded, and useless, you are at a major turning point in your life with some important choices to make. I recently heard someone say, in half jest and half truth, "Everyone knows that all a man needs to be happy is cable television and a couch." The couch serves a purpose and so does television, but if used to excess they are a dangerous combination.

You can lead a sedentary lifestyle, grow feeble and old as you wait to die, or you can make a fresh start at a new, meaningful life. You don't have to continue on a downhill slide to nowhere; you can begin right now to take charge of your new life away from the workplace. If you are fortunate, retirement can last for one-third of your life, so it's essential that you make that time as meaningful and fulfilling as possible.

When you were a vital part of the workforce you focused on goals associated with your career, making a living, and raising a family. Now you are at a new stage in life, in uncharted waters where nobody tells you what to do, you make the rules, and you decide your destination. They call it retirement, but does that mean you are obliged to play endless rounds of golf, game after game of tennis, or simply soak up the Florida sun? Of course not. Your brain still itches for a challenge, your body wants to keep moving, and your spirit seeks adventure. But you have to make it happen.

Being retired does not mean that you can no longer feel that old sense of achievement, satisfaction, and reward that you once had when you

---

🚶 Go for It!

If you happen to live alone, it's important to join a group or club where you can meet other people. And once you join a group, you should get actively involved by lending your support.

— Ethel Corbyn

42

were on the job. It simply means that you have to reorganize your new life so that you get that sense of fulfillment from other sources.

On the next few pages we explore your longevity in order to establish a solid base to work from. Once that is done we'll ask you to analyze your present situation in terms of physical activity and make a commitment to do *something* that will make your lifestyle a more active one. Now, have some fun with an activity that will take a peek at what the future has in store for you.

ACTIVITY # 2: YOUR TIMELINE

Before you embark on this activity, get comfortable at a desk or table with an 8.5" x 11" sheet of paper, a ruler, and pen or pencil. This should be an enjoyable few minutes, so take your time and relax as you reflect on the half century or more of your past, then focus on what lies ahead.

We will ask you to look back at your life and identify those significant events that made a difference to you and your family. Then you will be invited to explore your new life, from today onward to your Exit time. Let's get started, and the details will unfold as you proceed with the activity.

Follow the instructions below and keep an eye on the completed sample activity for Frank found on the next page.

Activity Instructions

1. Across the wide side of the page print your name and "Timeline."

2. Draw a heavy line under the "Timeline" heading, about two inches from the top, leave a margin of about one inch on each side.

3. On the far left of the line write "Enter" and on the far right side write "Exit." The word "exit" is just a delicate term for the year you leave this world.

4. On the left side below "Enter," fill in your year of birth.

5. About three-quarters of the way along the timeline draw a "You Are Here" sign to indicate where you are now and enter the current year.

6. Just above your timeline draw a line from "Enter" to "You Are Here" and enter your age.

7. Now, think about the significant events in your life and enter them in chronological order along your timeline between "Enter" and "You Are Here."

    Take a few minutes to think about your answers to this step. It's good idea to write out your thoughts and organize them on a separate sheet of paper before entering them on your timeline.

8. The sample timeline is intentionally brief and only shows the word "event" where you should enter your significant events such as your marriage, your son's birth, your daughter's graduation, etc. On your own timeline feel free to include all events and dates that have had a significant influence on your life.

Frank's Timeline

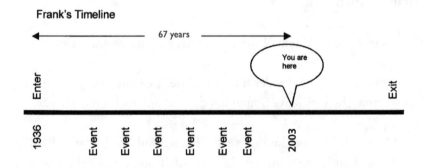

This Is Your Past

You have just taken a snapshot of your past with a few brief words to identify significant events that have shaped your life and that of those around you. This activity has allowed you to glimpse back over your shoulder. As you made your entries you must have thought about what might have been if you had taken a different turn at key stages of your life. But yesterday is gone and now it's time to live in the present and plan for the future. Like the rest of us, you are standing in the Exit line, waiting your turn, not knowing when that will be.

Our aim now is to help you estimate your life expectancy and decide how to make the best use of your future years. We live so much longer these days. Life expectancy at birth in Canada in 1999 was **76.3 years for males and 81.7 years for females**. In 1920–22 our life expectancy was only 59 years for males and 61 years for females. In Roman times, about 2,000 years ago, life expectancy at birth was a mere 25 years. We've come a long way.

Putting Your Life in Perspective

Like it or not, you know that most of your birthdays have already passed. In the future there will be fewer, but each one will be more precious than the last. We will help you determine approximately how many birthdays you have left, then help you establish your lifetime goals for the years between now and your Exit time. Sure, you may find it unpleasant to entertain thoughts about your own demise, but let's be realistic: it's inevitable, so why not take your best shot at determining how many years you have left. Once you have that number you will be in a better position to decide how you want to use that precious time.

Here's what to do:

1. On your timeline, draw a line with arrows at either end to depict your future life between "You Are Here" and "Exit." Make the line

somewhat thicker to indicate the importance of this period. See the sample timeline on the next page.

2. Based on family history, your health, and your lifestyle, make your best estimate of how many years you have from now until Exit. Take into account such factors as smoking, weight, stress, inactivity, diet, and how old your parents were when they died. When you have come up with your best estimate of how many years you have left, enter that number on your future years timeline. In our sample, we have estimated Frank's life expectancy at 79, therefore +12 years has been entered on his future timeline.

If you are on the Internet:

3. Let's get a second opinion about that number you arrived at. Life insurance actuaries constantly study longevity and the factors that impact our lifespan. As a result, their predictions about longevity are probably more accurate than most. So let's play the Longevity Game provided by Northwestern Mutual Life Insurance. Here's what to do if you have access to the Internet:

    Go to Northwestern's Web site at www.northwestern mutual.com. From the home page click on "Calculators," found on the "Learning Centre" drop menu, then from the list that appears click on "The Longevity Game." Answer all the questions and then enter the difference between the longevity prediction you get and your present age on your "future years" timeline.

Now you have two estimates of how many years you have left before your Exit time. Take a look at both numbers and choose which you think is the best estimate. There is no doubt that raw numbers about something as major as your Exit time can be shocking, but this exercise puts emphasis on the need to establish some very important goals for your remaining years.

Northwestern's Longevity game suggested that Frank would live to age 81, thus I have entered +14 years on the timeline.

Frank's Timeline

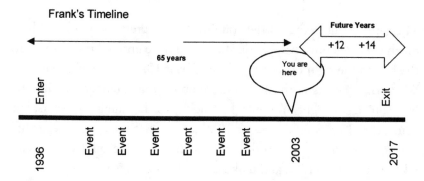

Did You Notice?

While making your entries on Northwestern's Longevity Game you may have noticed the factors built into their longevity analysis. Some of them were smoking, diet, exercise, weight, and stress. Do you recall that back on page three we began this book with reference to Dr. Feindel's three warnings to me:

1. Don't Smoke
2. Eat right
3. Exercise

If you are interested in good health and longevity it seems you just can't shake off those three fundamentals.

Did you also notice that under the Exercise category of the Longevity Game you gain years for being active? You gain six additional years for a "Very Active" response as compared to "Not Active." If you missed that, please return to the Longevity Game and click on each of the buttons: Very Active, Somewhat Active, and Not Active. Note that:

- when you click on Not Active you lose three years
- when you click on Somewhat Active you gain three years
- when you click on Very Active you gain another three years

How's that for a wake-up call to exercise!

It's Your Move

The genie is out of the bottle: you now have a pretty good idea of how much time you have before your Exit. You have entered the number in the box to the right of your timeline. Was it 10, 15, or maybe even 25? We know there is nothing definitive about that number, but it's the best you've got, right? You may be stuck with the number of years, but you can roll up your sleeves and influence what happens in your life during that time. You can drift along on automatic pilot or you can take charge of your life and make things happen. It's up to you.

Focus on Future Years

1. On a fresh sheet of paper draw a timeline to depict your future years similar to the chart shown below. On the left end of the timeline enter "I am here" and the year. On the right enter "Exit" and the year. Across the top, boldly enter the number of wonderful years before your Exit time.

    Ponder those future years for a while, for they represent the rest of your life. Your project for the next few minutes, hours, or even days is to think about how you want to spent your remaining years. Everything in this book is aimed at helping you get the most out of life from where you are now until your Exit time.

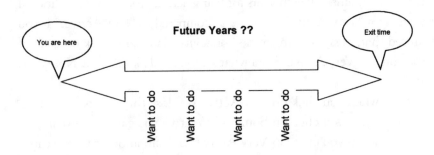

2. Here are a few suggestions that will help you identify what you may like to do in your future years:

    Talents: Make a list of your talents or abilities that make you unique as an individual. Natural talents can vary from music or athletic ability to a talent for working with people.

    Skills: Make a list of your skills or those things you have learned to do. Skills will range from carpentry to cooking, and from teaching to computing.

    Want to do: Many people can identify something they have always wanted to do but for one reason or another never got around to. Now is a good time make a list of those "want to do" yearnings. Many people find that retirement is an ideal time to begin a search of their ancestry. Others decide to volunteer, take up a hobby, or write their memoirs.

    Want to learn: Thousands of adults are attending evening or day classes to satisfy their desire to learn something new or pick up where they left off years ago. If you have such a longing now is the time to make a list. A retired friend of ours is now learning to play the bagpipes, something he just never had time to do before.

3. Once you have completed your four lists, select your best ideas and enter them in the space below where you can refer back to them at a later date. Try to be specific in your statements. Remember, nothing is cast in stone, so revisit your list and revise it once in a while.

What I want to do with
The Rest of My Life:

_____

_____

_____

_____

_____

_____

_____

ACTIVITY # 3: ARE YOU FIT ENOUGH TO ENJOY YOUR FUTURE?

Take a few minutes to analyze your lifestyle and determine whether you are active enough to keep fit as you grow older. Review your "Want to do" list and check off the items that require you to be in good physical condition. Will you be fit enough to do the things you want to do?

1. What type of exercise or physical activity do you do?

2. Do you engage in moderate physical activity for a minimum of 30 minutes, 4 days a week?

3. Is there a specific health improvement you would like to achieve through exercise? If so, what is it?

4. Six months from now what would you like to be able to do that you cannot do now? Be specific: i.e., walk three miles in one hour, climb five flights of stairs, etc.

Your Commitment to Health

Based upon what you learned in Chapter 1, and considering the activities in your "Want to do" list, you may be ready to begin taking better care of your body.

Remember, anything is better than nothing, and everyone has his or her own starting place. Without getting into details at this time, you may be ready to make a commitment to a more active lifestyle. If so, make that promise to yourself now by signing "My Commitment" below.

My Commitment
Yes, I want to improve my health and the quality of my life. Accordingly, I hereby make a commitment

to become more physically active in my future years. I will decide on the specifics of a program at the end of Chapter 4.

Signed _____ Date _____

Making It Happen

If you just made a commitment to your health, congratulations! Making a decision to change your lifestyle from inactive to active may be the most important step you have ever made. The important thing is to get started. Elainne says it this way:

Get into the swim of fitness, even if you start with the dog paddle.

— Elainne LaLanne

QUICK SUMMARY

- Make no mistake, active living is essential for health and quality of life.

- You now have an approximation of how many years you have between now and your Exit time. It is up to you to make the best use of that remaining time.

- If you signed "My Commitment" you have taken a crucial first step on the road to a happier lifestyle.

In this chapter:

- Get specific about the type of activity you want to try out.

- Identify your activity preference: solo, with a partner, or in a group.

- Learn about activity types: endurance, flexibility, and strength.

- Find out how to knock down the barriers and stay motivated.

The greatest health risk for older adults is sedentary living.
— World Health Organization, 1997

Your Commitment

In the previous chapter you made a commitment to become more physically active. If you follow through on that commitment your health will improve, you will have more energy, you will feel better about yourself, and you will have an improved outlook on life. You know the direction you want to take, so let us begin.

You are mentally prepared to get active, now here is your chance to decide exactly what activities you would like to try out. How about sky diving or mountain climbing? Just kidding, although plenty of folks over 50 do seek out that sort of daring activity. Some of our more adventurous friends have canoed the Nahanie River and the coast of Greenland, while others in search of a hiking challenge have trekked in such far away places as New Zealand, Bavaria, Costa Rica, Crete, Tuscany, Austria, and the Yellow Mountains of China.

Making the Change

Making a behavioral change seldom happens immediately. It takes time. Whether you are trying to quit smoking or change from an inactive to an active lifestyle, most people go through a series of steps before actually achieving success. It's not easy to break old habits, so don't be surprised if you encounter obstacles along the way. Your old sedentary voice will say, "You're too busy to exercise, you're too tired, you've got better things to do," but don't give in. Listen to your other voice, the one encouraging you to actually discover the best years of your life. Think about how good you will feel once you have turned the corner to a more active lifestyle.

Be aware that change takes place in stages and that it is normal to encounter setbacks as you move from one stage to the next. The key is to keep moving towards your goal of active living.

Take Your Pick

Later in this chapter we will ask you to consider your options and indicate your preferences for the following:

1. Select an activity: decide which ones you want to try out.
2. Select from activity types: endurance, flexibility, or strength.
3. Decide the setting: solo, with a partner, or in a group.

Read the chart for further explanation.

Fulfill your commitment to become more active		
Take your pick		
1 **Select Activity**	**2** **Identify Activity Type**	**3** **Decide the Setting**
There are dozens of activities to choose from. In the pages that follow we have suggested various activities ranging from walking to weightlifting, but there are many more sports and activities out there not shown in this book.	There are three general types of activities. In this chapter we introduce you to the three types and identify sports or activities that fit each type. Some activities fall under more than one type. **The types are:** **Endurance** **Flexibility** **Strength**	A third factor to consider when selecting your sport or activity is whether you would prefer to work out: **Solo** alone, that is With a **Partner** such as your spouse or a friend or in a **Group** or a ***Combination*** of all three.

1. Select Your Activities

Once you decide to get active, the next logical step is to decide what sport or activity you want to try that will give you the exercise you want. It is quite possible that you already know what you want to do. On the other hand, you may have no idea where to start. To help you out, we have prepared lists of activities later in this chapter. These lists are only suggested activities and not intended to be all-inclusive.

Here are a few guidelines to follow before selecting your activities. Choose activities that you have some familiarity with or that you feel confident you will enjoy. You want to have fun and enjoy your new active lifestyle, so don't get into something that you will find intimidating or that is too difficult to perform. Think back to a sport like skating, swimming, or cycling that you enjoyed as a kid. You may want to try the same thing again.

If you have not exercised for some time or if you're in poor shape, don't overdo it. Don't take on more than you can handle. Don't hesitate to start off by joining a group involved with one of the "gentle sports" like lawn bowling, yoga, or walking. By all means start off slowly with a modest goal that you will stick with. Select the time of the day that will fit best with your normal routine. It's better to choose one activity and stick with it than select two or three, then drop out before you have even worked up a sweat.

Several months after my heart surgery I spent the winter in Florida, but I continued walking four miles each morning. I remember quite vividly one particular day when it occurred to me that, in addition to the constant solo walking, I should search for an activity that would allow me to have interaction with other people. After a bit of mental brainstorming I recalled that I had at one time enjoyed a few canoe outings. As soon as I returned home I searched through the yellow pages, made several phone calls, and joined the canoe club that appealed to me most. I'm still an active member thirteen years later. Once you get the urge to do something in your best interests, follow through with the steps necessary to bring your idea to fruition.

 Go for It!

You must commit yourself. Join a gym or a community centre. Tell them what you want to accomplish. Pay for the first month and challenge them to keep you so satisfied that you will renew your membership.

— Stewart McTavish

2. Three Activity Types

The objective of these first chapters is to nudge inactive Canadians off the couch or pry them away from their computer long enough to spend a few minutes a day exercising their body. While we don't want to burden you with technicalities at this early stage, there seems to be no alternative. There are three general "types" of physical activity. The experts, as well as common sense, suggest that a good exercise program should contain a mix of activities from each of the following three categories:

- **Endurance** (aerobic) activities keep your cardiovascular system in good condition. Some examples are brisk walking, cycling, swimming, skating, and cross-country skiing. They all improve the health of your heart, lungs, and circulatory system.
- **Flexibility** (stretching) activities should be a part of any fitness plan. Tennis, curling, dancing, housework, tai chi, and yoga are some examples. Flexibility exercises keep you limber and even play a part in preventing falls.
- **Strength** (resistance) activities such as weight training build your muscles and make you stronger so you can do the normal lifting, carrying, pushing, and pulling required to get you through the day.

As you will see later in this chapter, when we list sample activities they are categorized according to one of the above types. Please be aware that many of these activities could easily fall under more than one group. Swimming for instance is listed as an endurance activity but it also does wonders as a flexibility exercise.

Throughout this book we tend to use the terms "physical activity" and "exercise" interchangeably, but there is a distinction. Here is how the Canadian Health Network describes these terms:

> **Physical activity** is defined as any bodily movement that burns up energy.

Exercise is a sub-category of physical activity. The difference here is that the movements are planned, structured, and repetitive. People who exercise do it to enhance or sustain their physical fitness.

3. Your Activity Setting

Early in your move to a more active lifestyle you should give thought to which setting you would prefer for your activities or workouts:

- **Solo**: doing your activities alone;
- **Partner**: doing your activities with your spouse or a friend;
- **Group**: doing your activities in a group, or as a member of a club; or
- Some **combination** of the above.

All of these factors have a bearing on whether you will enjoy your new world of fitness, and your level of enjoyment determines whether you continue to be active. Here are some of the pros and cons of each situation.

Solo

Some activities like gardening are best done alone. Hiking, walking, or cycling may be done solo, with a partner, or in a group. If you live in a condo you probably have access to a small gym and a swimming pool where you can exercise solo whenever you wish without having to concern yourself about others. One advantage of exercising alone is that you can pick your own time and place and enjoy privacy while exercising. But there are major disadvantages in setting out to exercise alone:

- You're more likely to lose interest and quit;
- You don't have an instructor's input on the correct way to perform an exercise; and

- You have no interaction with other people. If even a small part of your reason for becoming active was to have additional social contact, try to find that social contact in the activities you select.

Partner

If you have a spouse, a partner, or close friend, try to get him or her involved too. If your partner is not interested don't let that hold you back. Many men and women are extremely active in physical fitness activities while their spouses pursue some other endeavour. Don't deprive yourself of something you want to do just because your spouse has other interests. If your partner has never shown any interest in exercise and is emphatic about not wanting to become active, don't delay; look after your own health by becoming physically active on your own.

Group

There is energy in a group. Wherever you live there is probably a seniors' centre nearby that offers fitness classes similar to the ones identified later in this chapter. If you have never been involved in exercising or sports or "working out," or if you have been inactive for some time, this is an ideal place to begin. There is a certain enthusiasm generated within a group, and it's catching. You will work harder and longer in a group than you will alone. I am a firm believer in performing your activities within a group. Here are a few of the advantages of a group:

- By attending an instructor-led group exercise class you learn how to exercise. If you are not accustomed to exercising this is a must, for if exercises are not performed correctly they can do more harm than good;
- When you join a group exercise class it is usually a commitment of one or two days per week and you are more likely to attend; and

- Exercising is more fun when you are with a group.

If you get some of your exercise through a sport such as cycling, hiking, or canoeing, that sport takes on added value in a group. You still get your exercise, but you also have social contact with like-minded people. In a group there is always a fun atmosphere and a sense of sharing that adds to the pleasure of what you are doing.

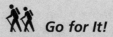 *Go for It!*

It's unlikely that anyone will knock on your door and invite you out, so visit your local community centre. Find out what's going on and what might be of interest to you.

— Ken Holden

Where to Look for Fitness Services

Check the Yellow Pages, your local city hall, and other sources of information in your community and you will be amazed at the variety of private and government organizations anxiously waiting to keep you fit and healthy.

In most communities you will find city-owned fitness centres, privately owned fitness clubs, seniors' centres, and the YMCA/YWCA. Most health clubs have a full range of facilities, including a large variety of treadmills, stepping machines, and stationary bikes. Some locations will have a swimming pool, squash courts, tennis courts, and a walking/jogging track. Many will also offer custom-designed exercise training, and many will include group fitness classes. Fitness supervisors at these facilities are graduates of recognized physical education programs. Costs will vary from just a few dollars a year at a seniors' centre to a few hundred at a private fitness club with more amenities than you will ever put to use.

Remember, you don't have join a fitness club to stay in shape — there are alternatives. You are not striving for bulging biceps, killer abs, or great glutes, you just want to stay physically fit. You can accomplish that by walking, hiking, or cycling a minimum of 30 minutes a day, 4 days a week.

Check It Out

Before joining a fitness centre, get a copy of its program and see what it has to offer. Talk to the staff and some of the members, and look over the facilities to see if the environment is right for you. Some clubs do not offer group fitness classes, so if that's what you are looking for, make sure it is included before you join. It's a good idea to visit a centre when a class is in session and observe the group in action. Members and staff will invariably make you feel at home, and if you join, you'll feel like an old pro in no time at all.

Low-impact group classes are designed for members who want to become more active. To jazz up the terminology you'll find some intriguing titles such as Stretch 'n Sweat, Stretch 'n Tone, and Young at Heart Fitness. The style and format will vary from one instructor to another, but they will usually be carried out to the beat of music and include the following sequence:

- a warm-up, moving around at an easy pace for several minutes;
- low-impact aerobics;
- muscular strength exercises using light weights to improve your muscle tone;
- stretching exercises to improve your joint movements and increase your range of motion and flexibility; and finally
- a cool-down.

Seniors' Centres

Call them what you will, there must be thousands of seniors' centres, community centres, recreation centres, and older adult centres across Canada that act as a gathering place for men and women age 55 or older. The Older Adult Centre in Mississauga may be typical of what happens across the country. It has a membership of over 1,500, a staff of 3, a volunteer board of directors, and 150 volunteers who attend to the daily operation of the facility.

Its schedule includes programs in education, recreation, health and wellness, and special events. All of this is available for a token membership fee and a small charge to take part in special programs.

There was a time when I discounted seniors' centres as a place where frail old folks shuffled from the bridge table to the bingo hall. But no more. The seniors' centres that I have visited offer a variety of top-notch fitness classes conducted by qualified instructors. They offer group fitness activities such as stretching, aerobics, line dancing, ballroom dancing, yoga, tai chi, and much more. I challenge anyone to attend a Sweat & Stretch session at the Older Adults Centre in Mississauga and not be impressed by the experience. The instructors put enthusiasm into their sessions and make you feel like a part of the group as you sweat and stretch your muscles from your neck down. Instructors don't force you to do more than you are capable of. On the contrary, they constantly caution participants not to overdo an activity and to stop at any time. You should know your own limitations, but your instructor will encourage you to heed the warnings of your body.

No doubt, many who attend seniors' centres across Canada confine their time to socializing and pursuing passive activities, but thousands more are physically active. If you are looking for physical activity that benefits your health you'll find it in spades at these centres. Give them a try.

Missing Part
By Dorothy Heller

I spent a fortune on a trampoline,
A stationary bike and a rowing machine,
Complete with gadgets to read my pulse,
And gadgets to prove my progress results,
And others to show the miles I've charted,
But they left off the gadget to get me started!

Selecting Your Activities

On the next few pages you will be asked to select one or more activities from the sample activities listed. Our purpose is to encourage you to get active by selecting an activity, trying it out, and eventually making it a part of what you do on a regular basis. As previously mentioned, these lists of activities are not meant to be all-inclusive. If you don't see the activity you are looking for on the list, simply add it.

Basically, there are two ways to get your exercise. You can work out in a gym (fitness centre) or you can get your exercise from a sport. Some people thrive on regular trips to the gym to maintain good health, while others get bored with the routine and quit exercising.

If the gym routine holds little appeal for you, search for a sport that will give you the exercise you need and put some fun into your life. You may get a lot more enjoyment from going for a walk, a hike, or a bike ride in the great outdoors than pacing on a treadmill indoors. If you get your exercise the fun way, doing something you enjoy, you will be more likely to stick with it.

Near the end of the chapter you will be asked to summarize your choices, so make your selections as you proceed through the next few pages.

Endurance (Aerobic) Activities

The Mayo Clinic Family Health Book describes an aerobic activity as one that requires your heart and lungs to function at an increased rate, supplying your cells with more oxygen (literally aerobic means "exercise with oxygen"). Your main exercise should be an aerobic exercise such as swimming, cycling, walking, skating, canoeing, cross-country skiing, or dancing. Numerous workout classes at seniors' centres and other clubs devote a significant part of their time to aerobic activity. These exercises will give you more energy and help your heart, lungs, and circulatory system.

Frequency

In its "Physical Activity Guide," Health Canada recommends a minimum of 30 minutes of moderate endurance exercises 4 days a week to benefit your health. What a bargain!

From the list below, check off the Endurance activities that you intend to incorporate into your exercise program. Then circle the appropriate letter — S, P, or G — to indicate whether you intend to perform the activity solo, with a partner, or in a group.

Sample Endurance (Aerobic) Activities

❑ Canoeing	S	P	G
❑ Cross-country skiing	S	P	G
❑ Cycling	S	P	G
❑ Dancing	S	P	G
❑ Fitness classes with aerobics	S	P	G
❑ Golf (no cart)	S	P	G
❑ Hiking	S	P	G
❑ Hockey seniors	S	P	G
❑ Kayaking	S	P	G
❑ Rowing	S	P	G
❑ Skating (ice)	S	P	G
❑ Skating (roller)	S	P	G
❑ Swimming	S	P	G
❑ Tennis	S	P	G
❑ Walking (briskly)	S	P	G
❑ Other: _____	S	P	G

Flexibility (Stretching) Activities

Stretching or flexibility exercises prevent muscles from becoming short and tight. Activities such as bowling, yoga, curling, tennis, and dancing all help to stretch your muscles. Stretching exercises should become an important component of your fitness program.

You can do stretching exercises at home or in a group setting. Since there are important dos and don'ts associated with stretching, you should learn how to stretch from a qualified fitness instructor before doing it on your own. Once you have learned the techniques of stretching you can establish your own routine and stretch at home. There are a number of good books on stretching. My favourite reference book is *Stretching* by Bob Anderson. The illustrations are clear and the book is divided into useful categories that describe the appropriate stretching routines to follow before and after such activities as cycling, hiking, and others. Anderson also provides specific stretching recommendations for those over 50.

Frequency

Stretch for about 10 minutes, 4 to 7 days a week. Stretching exercises will go a long way toward preventing cramps and stiffness. If you are troubled with back problems, seek the advice of a health professional and you will find that certain stretching exercises can be highly beneficial for your back.

Stretch Out in the Garden

Yes, gardening is a popular physical activity for Canadian adults. In fact, it ranks up there with walking, and it's easy to see why. Gardening is an exercise that allows you to combine fresh air and sunshine with enjoyable, productive work. While you do all that digging, planting, weeding, watering, and raking you strengthen your arm and leg muscles and build strong bones.

But yard work is physically demanding, so ease into it at the start of a season so you don't strain your back and shoulder muscles. If you don't have a garden of your own, you may want to check out other options such as joining a group of gardening volunteers. Most communities have such groups who tend to the gardens at such places as seniors' homes.

From the list below, check off the Flexibility activities that you intend to incorporate into your exercise program. Then circle the appropriate letter — S, P, or G — to indicate whether you intend to perform the activity solo, with a partner, or in a group.

Sample Flexibility Activities

❏ Bowling	S	P	G
❏ Curling	S	P	G
❏ Dancing	S	P	G
❏ Fitness classes with stretching	S	P	G
❏ Gardening	S	P	G
❏ Golf	S	P	G
❏ Housework	S	P	G
❏ Lawn Bowling	S	P	G
❏ Stretching exercises	S	P	G
❏ Tai Chi	S	P	G
❏ Tennis	S	P	G
❏ Volleyball	S	P	G
❏ Yoga	S	P	G
❏ Other: _____	S	P	G

Strength (Resistance) Activities

These exercises will strengthen your muscles and help your bones stay strong. Without regular use, muscles can become flabby, soft, and weak. At first glance you may think that any reference to muscles and strength should be confined to body builders at a sweaty gym, but that's not so. If you decide to cycle you need strength to peddle your bike, if you decide to take up canoeing you need strength to paddle. And I'm sure you want to be able to carry your own luggage on your next trip. Yes, muscles are needed for everyday living so don't let yours deteriorate. The old saw still applies, "If you don't use it you'll lose it."

Instructor-led workouts at seniors' centres, community centres, and other locations may use hand and ankle weights or rubber bands to pro-

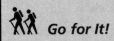

Go for It!

Associate with active people.
— John Galbraith

vide strength-training exercises. They usually incorporate a healthy mix of all three activity categories during a one-hour group session. A typical one-hour session may be: 10 minutes for warm-up, 30 minutes for the main aerobic activity, with the final 20 minutes allocated to strength activities, stretching, and cool-down. By joining such a group you are sure to get the recommended balance of the three activity groups.

Frequency

Two to four days a week. Weight-training specialists state that you should always allow 48 hours between weight-training workouts to allow your muscles to fully rest and recover.

Weight Training for Strength

As a member of the 50-plus group you may find the thought of weight training or strength training a bit scary. For many of us, the gym is unfamiliar territory and the idea of struggling to push, pull, or lift an apparatus that would prefer to remain at rest can be terrifying. But don't run for cover just yet. Your apprehension is probably nothing more than a fear of the unknown.

Most of us associate strength training with the world of bulging muscles and bodybuilding. That's yesterday's vision. Today, strength or weight training is considered an integral part of most well-balanced fitness programs. Research shows that by the time we reach the age of 55 or 60 we will have lost about half of our strength and muscle mass. Strength training helps our muscles remain strong and active.

Special weight-training courses for older adults are now being offered in many fitness centres across the country. Not too long ago Olga and I enrolled in a group weight-training course for older adults in Mississauga. The training consisted of two, one-hour sessions each week for five weeks.

Our group was assigned a qualified personal trainer, and we thoroughly enjoyed the experience as we learned how to use each piece of exercise equipment. There was absolutely nothing intimidating about working out in the gym with dozens of like-minded men and women striving to achieve the same goal. In your search for ways to stay fit, consider adding weight training to your repertoire of activities to choose from.

From the list below, check off the Strength activities that you intend to incorporate into your exercise program. Then circle the appropriate letter — S, P, or G — to indicate whether you are going to perform this activity solo, with a partner, or in a group.

Sample Strength Activities

❑ Thera Band stretching exercises you can do at home	S P G
❑ Climbing stairs	S P G
❑ Fitness classes with strength activities	S P G
❑ Heavy yard work	S P G
❑ Weightlifting	S P G
❑ Other: _____	S P G

Range of Effort

In the world of physical activity or exercise you will often find the terms very light, light, moderate, vigorous, and maximum used to describe the amount of effort or work required to carry out a variety of activities.

As you know from the first chapter, in order to benefit your health you should perform activities at the moderate effort level. Health Canada's Physical Activity Guide recommends a minimum of 30 minutes of moderate activity 4 days per week.

So how much effort is considered to be moderate effort? The chart below provides you with a visual yardstick. Moderate effort is a brisk walk, which calls for more effort than bowling, but less effort than cross-country skiing.

◄───────────────► **Range of Effort or Exertion** ────────────►

Very Light Effort	Light Effort	Moderate Effort	Vigorous Effort	Maximum Effort
Strolling	Light walking Bowling Golf on foot	Brisk walking Cycling Line Dancing	Jogging Cross-country skiing Aerobics	Sprinting Racing

A minimum of 30 minutes of <u>moderate activity</u> 4 days per week will benefit your health.

Make It a Way of Life

Although we have focused on specific activities or exercises during this chapter, don't lose sight of the fact that your goal is to make active living a way of life. Don't be limited to performing a few specific activities according to a designed performance schedule. A few years ago, when speaking to a young woman who jogged 30 minutes every morning before breakfast, I asked, "How do you maintain the motivation to keep at it every day?" She responded, "Jogging is just as much a part of my morning routine as brushing my teeth." That's the way we should look at active living. It should become as natural as any other part of our daily life.

Here are a few examples of what we mean by active living as a way of life.

- When you park at a shopping mall, don't search for the spot nearest the entrance; park where you are forced to walk a couple minutes to the mall entrance.
- If you live in a condo or apartment, don't always use the elevator. Take the stairs once in a while. Joe, a hiking friend, told me this story that indicates how far we still have to go before active living becomes a way of life:

Joe works on the third floor of an old office building with an antiquated elevator that constantly breaks down and even traps people between floors. To avoid this frustration, and because he's an active fellow, Joe always walks up and down the three flights of stairs. One day when a co-worker complained about the elevator, Joe said to her, "Maggie, I have the perfect solution for you. Avoid the aggravation of the elevator altogether by taking the stairs like I do. It will even be good for you."

She looked at him in disbelief and said, "No thanks!" There's no doubt about it: active living as a way of life is not just around the corner.

- In the subway or shopping mall, take the stairs instead of the escalator.
- If you live in a house, do your own gardening and cut your own lawn.
- Don't always drive your car for those short trips to the corner store. Wear your runners and walk instead, but walk briskly so you get some health benefit out of it.
- Wash your car by hand.
- If you normally get around by bus, get off a couple of stops early and walk the rest of the way. Again, walk briskly.
- If you normally drive your car to a subway parking lot and then take the subway to your destination, try parking your car a few blocks from the subway, then walk those few blocks.

Here's an incident from the travel section of a national newspaper that confirms that active living is not a normal part of our thinking. In describing a specific trip, the travel writer mentioned there was considerable hiking and walking involved. She concluded by suggesting that potential participants take it easy and get plenty of rest in preparation for the active weeks that lay

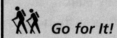 **Go for It!**

Establish a set routine for your exercise or activity and do it even if you don't feel like it. I usually go for a brisk walk or a bike ride in the morning even though I have to talk myself into it. I always feel great when I get back.

— Cato Bayens

ahead. It would have made much more sense for the travel writer to have said, "Start getting in shape now before the trip, not during the trip." That way the participants would have built up their muscles and endurance levels before leaving.

Get Up 'n Go in the Cardiac Wing

At this point, I want to discuss the advantages of instructor-led exercises by relating my own experience as a member of a group. Hopefully, this account will minimize any concerns you may have that physical activity will result in injury or pain, or that it won't do you any good. This description will also point out the need for medical approval before beginning an exercise program.

After my heart bypass surgery, I joined the cardiac wing of the Toronto Rehab Centre headed by Dr. Terry Kavanagh. The centre is equipped with an indoor track, various exercise equipment, and a staff of medical technicians. Following a thorough evaluation I was given what they called an "exercise prescription" — a statement of the exercise I was expected to complete at that time. Although I attended the centre only twice each week I was expected to complete my walking prescription at home on the remaining days. On the days I did my walking at the centre, a staff member checked my pace, my pulse, and my blood pressure periodically during my workout. I started out slowly and gradually built up my pace and distance. As a result, I received a new exercise prescription periodically throughout my rehabilitation.

I still have copies of two prescriptions. Note that the prescriptions state the distance as well as the speed I was expected to walk. Here they are:

- **Three months after surgery:** Walk 1 mile in 18 minutes, 5 times per week.
- **Fifteen months after surgery:** Walk 4 miles in 60 minutes, 5 times per week.

Note the difference in these two prescriptions:

- The first prescription, three months after surgery, called for only a one-mile walk five times a week.
- The second prescription called for a four-mile walk five times a week at a faster pace of four-miles per hour (not kilometres). That's what I was expected to do fifteen months after open-heart surgery.

> **Go for It!**
>
> Join a club. If you're like me, when you ski, canoe, or hike you want to be with other people.
> — Ray Crites

Let me emphasize that I was following a walking program prescribed by medical experts; there are thousands following similar programs in cardiac rehab centres across Canada. As you can see, it is through physical activity (exercise) that medical professionals help their heart patients put their lives back together again. They don't pamper their heart patients, they give them challenging workouts within a medically supervised environment, and it produces positive results.

After my heart surgery, I did well for ten active years until a blocked blood vessel led to hospitalization. A medical team soon performed the angioplasty procedure, inserted the famous stent, and got my blood flowing freely again. To get back into shape and recover from that setback I enrolled in the Credit Valley Hospital Cardiovascular Rehab Program in Mississauga. Once more, under the direction of exercise specialists and health professionals, I found myself in a program that included walking, stretching, strengthening, and aerobic exercises. As the name implies, cardiac rehab programs are designed to help cardiac patients get back to normal after hospitalization or surgery. It has been my experience that the staff at cardiac rehab facilities are dedicated, taking a personal interest in each participant, and do a great job at guiding rehabilitation.

Thus after several months in a rehab program, patients are expected to use their own initiative to select a facility or devise a plan for keeping fit. In this book we help you do that. But bear in mind:

> For most people, exercising at a moderate intensity is safe. However, those who have a pre-existing condition such as heart disease or diabetes should consult

71

with their physician before embarking on an exercise program of moderate intensity.

Only 10 Percent Participate in Rehab

Following is an excerpt from a press release from the Cardiac Care Network, Toronto, July 15, 2001:

> Cardiovascular disease is one of the leading causes of death in Canada. An estimated 100,000 people in Ontario are living with heart disease. Research confirms that cardiac rehabilitation services can increase a cardiac patient's lifespan, improve the chances of returning to work, improve their quality of life, and lower the amount of medical treatment needed in the years to come.

The press release goes on to say that:

> In Ontario, over 8,000 patients participated in a cardiac rehabilitation program in 1999–2000 but those patients only represented 10 percent of the eligible cardiac population that would benefit from such a service.

It is difficult to understand how a cardiac patient who has visited death's door could pass up an opportunity to participate in a rehab program that virtually ensures increased longevity and a healthier lifestyle. Yet, the above data shows that an overwhelming majority of cardiac patients do just that. In 1995–96 there were more than 18,000 bypass surgeries and almost 24,000 angioplasties performed in Canada.

Other Special Programs

Special physical activity programs are also available for those with special needs, such as patients with osteoporosis, Parkinson's disease, multiple sclerosis, stroke survivors, and others. I have observed the osteoporosis program in action and it's a gentle one that includes walking, light cardiovascular stretching, and weight-bearing exercises that promote flexibility, reduce muscle tension, and increase bone density.

How to Stay Motivated

In Chapter 1 we identified a dozen or more reasons or excuses people find for not remaining active. You may remember that some of the barriers we discussed were lack of time, lack of willpower, health problems, fatigue, and financial considerations. By now, we hope you have resolved those issues and are prepared for some positive suggestions of how to keep motivated.

It's easy to get lazy, miss a few days or weeks and eventually stop altogether. Your challenge now is to remain committed to your activity program for an extended period of time. Here is a list of techniques you can use that will help you stick with it. Select a few that will work for you and use them.

Make It a Rule: Exercise Comes First

- Using a highlighter, mark up your calendar to indicate the time of the day and days of the week for your activity. As you mark your calendar, mentally tell yourself that these days are set aside for your exercise program, that they are "taken" and only an emergency will you allow you to deviate from your plan.
- Despite the above comment, be flexible. If you would like to change the time of day or days of the week you work out, go ahead and do it. If you would like to switch from walking to cycling, do that, too. Your goal is stay fit and have fun at the same time.
- Place a reminder note about your activity days on the fridge.

- Tell your friends and family about your new-found regular activities. It's normal to quietly think, "I'm not going to tell anyone in case I quit." That's a mistake. You are looking for ways to stay motivated, and telling others is one way to ensure that you will stick with your plan. Six months from now you can boast that you are still working out with the Stretch 'n Sweat group.
- Keep a record of your activities. Buy a small book. Call it your "activity book" and use it exclusively to record everything associated with your activities.
- If you live in Ontario, contact Active Ontario and ask for one of its 42-day laminated "Stick To It" wall posters, which will enable you to check off activities on your exercise program.
- Use a coloured marker to check off the date on a calendar every time you complete an activity.
- The Bruce Trail Hiking Association publishes a small book containing a series of detailed maps showing various sections of the Bruce Trail. Whenever I hiked a section of the trail, I recognized my accomplishment by marking the hiked portion of the trail with a coloured highlighter, then I entered the date of the hike and the name of the leader. Most of us need these small rewards to keep going. If you do something significant like pulling someone out of a blazing fire, you will probably get a plaque from the mayor at a public ceremony, but in the meantime, while waiting for the big event, devise your own methods of getting recognition.
- If for some reason you miss a couple of activity sessions, don't beat yourself up about it. Focus on getting back into your routine again. That's what counts.
- There will often be times when you simply don't feel like doing your regular physical activity. Be aware that we all get that same feeling from time to time. We accept the slightest excuse to justify staying home rather than go on the walk, the hike, or the bike ride. Unless you are ill, don't give in to

your feelings of apathy or laziness. Muster up all the willpower you can, then get out there and do what you know will make you feel great.

- Constantly remind yourself of the rewards that lie ahead. Soon you will be in better condition, the consistent exercise will improve your overall health, you will have more energy, you will feel better, and you will look forward to your next activity outing.

- Give yourself a small reward every time you take part in an activity session or go for a walk or a cycling outing. Your reward can be something as simple as telling yourself you did well. If you feel better about yourself, have more energy, and feel more cheerful make a note of it in your activity book. One instructor I know ends each group activity session by leading the group in a round of loud applause. When I first saw this outburst of applause and cheering I wondered what was going on, but I soon realized that everyone was silently saying, "Hey, we did good and we feel great."

- Associate with other active, like-minded people.

- Have fun.

ACTIVITY # 4: SUMMARY OF ACTIVITIES SELECTED

1. Refer back to the pages where you checked off the activities that appealed to you.

2. Enter these activities on the worksheet below. Also indicate whether you prefer to carry out your activities solo, with a partner, or in a group.

Activity Summary				
Type	**Activities**	**Solo**	**Partner**	**Group**
Endurance				
Flexibility				
Strength				
Motivation	Name two techniques you will use to keep motivated. 1._____ 2._____			

Congratulations

All you have to do now is make it happen. Mark your calendar so you will know at a glance which days are reserved exclusively for your activity. Don't let anything else interfere with your appointments for health. Get into the habit of thinking about your activity every day. When you go to bed at night, remind yourself that tomorrow is "activity day." When you get up in the morning remind yourself again. Don't think of your activity as a negative thing; think of it as a positive addition to your lifestyle, something you enjoy doing, something you are doing for yourself, possibly the best thing you have done in years.

When you are out there swimming, hiking, walking, biking, or doing the sweat and stretch thing, working your muscles and breathing hard, remind yourself that you are doing what you only dreamed of doing in the past. You're chalking up health benefits and you'll keep coming back for more.

Don't Put It Off

If your selected activity requires attending a group class but the start date is not for a few weeks, don't lie around inactive in the meantime. Use your imagination, choose another secondary activity such as walking, and get going immediately while you are motivated and ready to get turned on.

QUICK SUMMARY

- Whatever your exercise program, it should include the three types of activities: endurance, flexibility, and strength.

- You will find energy in a group and get support from a partner.

- Active living is a way of life. Don't limit yourself to performing a few exercises according to a specific timetable.

- Staying motivated is a key component to active living. Find out what works for you and use it.

In this chapter:

- Learn the value of goal-setting and key guidelines to follow.

- Learn how to identify the steps that contribute to a goal.

- Write your own physical activity goal.

- Determine the steps that will turn your goal into a reality.

Don't wait for a light to appear at the end of the tunnel, stride down there and light the bloody thing yourself.

— Sara Henderson

He Shoots! He Scores!

Foster Hewitt, the legendary hockey broadcaster, coined the phrase, "He shoots! He scores!" way back in 1923 when he was a 21-year-old rookie. When he first voiced that famous phrase he was broadcasting an Ontario Hockey Association playoff game between Kitchener and Parkdale. Later, when Maple Leaf Gardens opened its doors in 1931, Hewitt sat in the gondola above the ice, and his distinctive voice flowed over the airwaves with a play-by-play description of Canada's favourite game. And that's the way it was every Saturday night for the next three decades.

When Foster Hewitt shouted, "He shoots! He scores!" he was of course referring to the fact that a player had taken aim, shot the puck towards the opponent's net, past the goalie, and into the net. If the puck found its mark, the player scored a goal. Scoring goals is not easily accomplished in any sport, but it's the primary purpose of the game and everyone on the team knows it. Every action taken on the ice is in some way intended to help score goals, or to prevent the opposing team from scoring. The objective of the game is clear: score goals.

If you spent your career in the business world you are well aware that goals are used in a similar manner to provide purpose and direction to successful companies and their employees. But it doesn't stop there. Goals are also required in your personal life. If you don't have goals in your life you may find yourself aimlessly wandering in any direction.

Lifetime Goals

Most of us don't spend much time thinking about our goals. We accept what comes our way and move with the flow wherever it takes us. Seldom do we stop to think that we can in fact control our time and our life if we want to. To do that we must first know what we want out of life and what direction we want it to take. That means setting goals and establishing priorities.

At this point we want to introduce the concept of goals and the need to establish goals in several key areas of your life. As I contemplate such a formidable task I'm reminded of the elephant story. Apparently a young man asked an older, wiser man, "How do you eat an elephant?" The wise old man replied, "One bite at a time." So, we'll proceed in bite-size steps as we help you establish your personal goals.

Setting goals is simply a matter of clearly pinpointing exactly what you hope to achieve and getting it down on paper. On the surface that sounds easy enough, but once you actually begin the task you may find it more

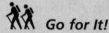 **Go for It!**

Join a club that's active or become a volunteer doing something you like to do. The first club I belonged to was a hiking club called the Pickering Plodders. They really got me moving and I have remained active ever since.

Find someone to join you in walks, hikes, a movie, or trips to the zoo. Whatever you do, you'll find it fulfilling.

— Joan Duncan

difficult than you originally expected. The problem is that most people do not have a clear vision of what they want out of life, so getting it down on paper may require considerable reflection.

Goals are not cast in stone; they reflect your best judgment today and they should be subject to change and revision as your life changes. Setting lifetime goals will cause you to focus on what you really want and steer you in the direction of a more fulfilling life. Once you know what you want you can go after it and make it happen. As someone once said, *Being clear about what you want and need is the first step in attaining it.*

Seek Balance in Your Life

There are at least six areas of your personal life in which you should consider establishing goals. Some authorities suggest seven categories, others say eight and even ten. We'll settle for six. But first, let's have a meeting of the minds on what a goal actually is. In my training days with Imperial Oil, I often worked with groups of people as we developed, discussed, and argued the topic of objectives and goals for hours on end, but there is no need for a prolonged discussion here. All we need is one definition of a goal for purposes of this book, and here it is:

> A goal is a clear, concise statement of an end result or desired outcome.

Although not always practised, it has long been recognized that we need balance in our lives. In hindsight, some of us now realize that years ago we allowed our jobs and careers to take precedence over the needs of our families. In more recent years attitudes have changed for the better and employers now recognize the need for a more balanced lifestyle. Thus we need to pursue more than one or two goals if we want to achieve balance in our lives. We all know people whose only goal appears to be the pursuit of money, while others with bulging muscles may have a singular goal of fitness. It's easy to fall into the trap of concentrating on one or two goals to the exclusion of all others. Almost unconsciously, we make adjustments to our goals as we go through life, piling one decade on top of another. Many years ago, one of your most important goal categories may have been career, but now that you are older, career is no longer on the front burner. The six categories that probably concern you most now are: education, family, finances, fitness & health, social & pleasure, and spirituality. As you read this book you may want to consider which goal categories your various activities involve. An awareness of these categories can help you achieve a balanced lifestyle.

Why Set Goals?

In Chapter 2 you arrived at an approximation of the number of years you have left between now and your Exit time. You may want to turn back to that chapter for another look at the number you so boldly entered on the future years timeline. Our purpose in taking you back is to remind you that when we speak of goals in this chapter, we are talking about your goals for your remaining years. Whether your lucky number was 10, as my son suggested for me, or 25 or more, any goals you set from now on apply to the enjoyment of your future years. There is no turning back.

Setting goals will help you pinpoint what you want to achieve during your remaining years. Once you know what you want to accomplish in each of the key areas of life you can go after it.

Goal-Setting Guidelines

Here's a second look at our definition of a goal: A goal is a clear, concise statement of an end result or desired outcome.

1. Put Your Goals in Writing
Once you write a goal on a sheet of paper or enter it into your computer you create a contract with yourself and set a process in motion that helps you carry through. Furthermore, by putting your goals in writing you clarify your thoughts and arrive at a precise statement of what you want to accomplish.

2. Personalize Your Goals

Your goals must belong to you and no one else. They must be goals that you want to achieve for your own reasons. There is no point in writing a goal that you don't believe in. That does not mean that you cannot share in the accomplishment of a larger, broader goal established by someone else. For instance, in August 1997, the federal and provincial/territorial ministers responsible for fitness, recreation, and sport set a collective goal to decrease by 10 percent the number of inactive Canadians by the year 2003. If you set a personal goal to become more physically active during that time period and you reach your goal, you will also contribute to Health Canada's goal and that's great. But your goal is still your personal goal.

3. Make Your Goals Measurable

A written goal statement must include such things as dates, times, and amounts so that your achievement (or lack of it) can be measured. If you write a goal statement about becoming more physically active and don't include a start date, you have not made a precise commitment to action, because any time will be okay.

Health Canada has told us quite clearly that we should accumulate a minimum of 30 minutes of moderate physical activity 4 days a week. Using slightly different words, that's what its "Physical Activity Guide for Older Adults" states. Health Canada is precise in its expectations of number of days per week and minutes of exercise per day, and you should be, too. Otherwise, you have no way to measure what you have accomplished.

Have you ever been in a situation like this? You say to your spouse, "Okay I'll pick you up at the corner of Portage and Main." You arrive at the northeast corner of that intersection two hours later, and your spouse is nowhere to be found. That's because she's been pacing back and forth at the southwest corner of Portage and Main for the past hour and a half. When you made arrangements to meet each other, the specifics of time and place were missing from the conversation. You assumed one thing, your spouse assumed another. It's the same thing with goal-setting: mean what you say and state it clearly.

4. Make Your Goals Realistic

Try not to set your goals based on your best performance of 20 years ago. Be realistic by taking into account your present age and your health. If you are not sure, consult with your health care professional. Don't set your goals so high that there is no hope of achieving them, for then you are sure to fail, and that's no fun. Once you know your level of performance you can strive to exceed your goals by, let's say, 10 percent. And remember you can always revise your goals.

Write Your Own Goal Statement

Assume you have been a cigarette smoker for most of your life and finally something has prompted you to seriously consider quitting. The more you think about it, the more convinced you are that every cigarette you smoke is another nail in your coffin. You want to quit as soon as possible but you know you can't quit cold turkey. Let's say you decided to stop smoking through a process of gradual withdrawal.

Okay, take your best shot at writing your Stop Smoking goal statement in the box below. Here is a reminder of our definition of a goal. A goal is a clear, concise statement of an end result or desired outcome. As you prepare your goal statement keep the four guidelines in mind: write it down, make it personal, make it measurable, and make it realistic. One final thought — focus only on the goal, not on how you are going to attain it. That's a separate issue. In other words, do not confuse setting your goal with reaching your goal.

My Stop Smoking Goal:

If you really are a smoker, you are writing a real goal. If so, good luck. Here are some suggestions that will help make stop smoking a reality for you.

Tips on How to Achieve This Goal — Or Any Goal

- Print your goal in large letters and make several copies of it. Post a copy on the fridge, in your office, in your car, and every other place you frequent.
- Visualize your completed goal; that is, visualize yourself at work, in your car, and at home without a cigarette in your mouth or in your hand.
- Think about yourself without any desire for a cigarette, free from that worry, free from the constant guilt, free from the ongoing concern about doing something that is bad for your health.
- Think about the positive aspects of not smoking every night before you go to bed and every morning when you awake.

If you presently smoke 40 cigarettes a day and you gave yourself forty days to gradually stop by withholding one cigarette each day, you will be a non-smoker on the fortieth day. If you write your goal today, and the date is May 21, you should stop smoking on June 30 of this year. With that in mind your goal statement would look like this:

Stop Smoking Goal
Date: May 21

Stop smoking by June 30 this year.

The above statement says that you will stop smoking 40 days from May 21. The goal is in writing, it is personal, measurable, and realistic.

The Calendar Example

Buy a special calendar for your Stop Smoking project, and at the end of each day enter the number of cigarettes you did not smoke that day. On the first day you enter "one" the second day you enter "two" and so forth. On the fortieth day you enter "forty," and you are now a non-smoker. This process gives you a reward every day as you tell yourself and indicate on the calendar that you are moving a little closer to your goal. The record on your calendar would look something like this:

Mon	Tues	Wed	Thurs	Fri	Sat	Sun
	Assume this is May 20th	21 1 cigarette not smoked	22 2 cigarettes not smoked	23 3 cigarettes not smoked	24 4 cigarettes not smoked	25 5 cigarettes not smoked
26 6 cigarette not smoked	27 7 cigarette not smoked	28 8 cigarette not smoked	29 9 cigarettes not smoked	30 10 cigarettes not smoked	31 11 cigarettes not smoked	and so on

Think up other rewards. Always have rewards to show yourself that you are making progress by getting closer to your goal. Avoid all negative self-talk and replace it with positive self-talk. Visualize your dream of not smoking, think about that wonderful life without a cigarette. That's how you help make it happen.

Focus on the Goal

A moment ago when you were about to prepare a goal statement we encouraged you to focus on the goal, not on how you are going to get there. This is an important aspect of goal-setting and deserves some elaboration. First you set your goal and *then* you decide how you are going to accomplish it.

Create Steps to Achieve Your Goal

Goal-Setting Sequence A-B-C-D

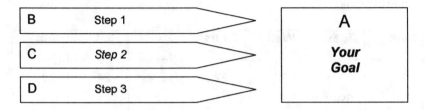

You may say, "If we worked on the steps first we would be in a better position to decide what the goal should be." At first glance that sounds logical enough, but think again: how can you work on the steps toward the accomplishment of a goal if you don't know what the goal is?

Stop Smoking Steps

The preceding tips are essentially steps to be taken in support of the Stop Smoking goal you prepared earlier, but they can be easily modified to suit any goal. Here's how these tips may appear if they were laid out as a sequence of steps.

The Steps

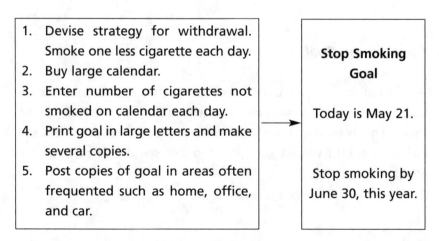

6. Think about positive aspects of not smoking every night and every morning.
7. Frequently visualize yourself not smoking.
8. Avoid negative self-talk and replace it with positive self-talk.

Marilyn Bell Conquers Lake Ontario

Imagine the preparation necessary to support 16-year-old Marilyn Bell's 52-kilometre, 21-hour swim across Lake Ontario on September 9, 1954. Marilyn's goal was to "Swim Lake Ontario from Youngstown, N.Y. to Toronto, Ontario," and she did. Some 250,000 people jammed the shores of Toronto's exhibition grounds to greet her and cheer her on as she swam ashore at about dusk. Think of all the steps necessary to make that goal a reality. But first, she set the goal:

Swim across Lake Ontario

Marilyn's goal was not:

Go for a swim in Lake Ontario, or
Swim across Lake Ontario if the waves don't get too high, or
Swim across Lake Ontario if I don't get too tired.

Now you know how to establish a goal. Good luck in your upcoming activity.

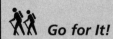

Go for It!

When you are accomplishing something you will feel good about it. The doing and pursuing is vital. Find out what appeals to you and get started.

— Bea Parkes

Where Have We Been?

Before completing your Physical Activity Goal, please take a few minutes to review what you have covered.

a) How Much Activity?

Briefly review Chapter 1 to remind yourself of Health Canada's physical activity recommendations in terms of level of activity, minutes per day, and days per week.

b) My Commitment

Turn back to Chapter 2, where you made a commitment to improve your health and quality of life. If you did not sign and date that commitment when you read Chapter 2, you may wish to do so now.

c) Summary of Your Chosen Activities

Turn back to Chapter 3. Take a few minutes to review your summary of the activities you want to try out. Also review the motivational techniques you intend to use to keep yourself going.

Food for Thought

In a moment we will ask you to complete Activity #5, Your Physical Activity Goal. When you put the words together for your goal statement, remember that you are speaking about an activity goal that you wish to attain at some time in the near future, not tomorrow. How long into the future will depend on your present physical condition, how much activity you do now, and possibly on what your doctor recommends.

When we prepared a goal statement for the Stop Smoking example the goal was to "stop smoking," but not for another 40 days. It was assumed that it would take 40 days for a smoker to become mentally and physically ready to stop that behaviour. There is always a series of steps or a process to go through before attaining any goal.

ACTIVITY # 5: YOUR PHYSICAL ACTIVITY GOAL

This is not a practice exercise, this is the real thing. You are about to complete your own personal Physical Activity Goal that will directly influence the rest of your life. Complete it with care, for you are dealing with your enjoyment of life.

In the Goal Worksheet on the next page we have allowed space for five steps, but please do not feel restricted by that number. Add as many or as few steps as you wish to get the job done. Sit back and think for a moment about the activities or sports that appeal to you, then think of the preparations you have to make to get started.

Instructions

1. Within the box headed "Physical Activity Goal," write out your physical activity goal.

2. In the boxes under the heading "Steps," identify the steps you will take to ensure that you accomplish your goal.

Goal Worksheet

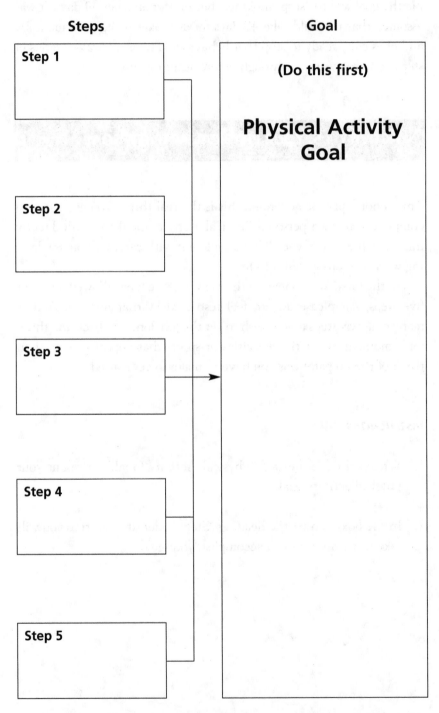

Steps   **Goal**

Step 1

(Do this first)

**Physical Activity
Goal**

Step 2

Step 3

Step 4

Step 5

Sara's Goal Worksheet

Here is Sara's worksheet showing her Physical Activity Goal and her steps for achieving it.

Step 1
Take a walk along River Road at least four days a week. Start with 15 minutes, then increase my walking time by 5 minutes each week until I reach 30 minutes, 4 days a week.

Step 2
I must find a partner soon. I know some friends who may like to join me in my quest for a healthier lifestyle. A partner will help me stick with it.

Step 3
Become better informed about the health benefits of regular exercise. Find out what's available in my own community in the area of activities, both physical and social. The better informed I am, the better my chances of keeping it up.

Step 4
Investigate further, then decide upon one of the sports that appealed to me. Right now, I favour the idea of joining a volleyball group.

(Do this first)

Physical Activity Goal

This is April 1st.

To be taking a brisk 30-minute walk at least 4 days a week by the fourth week in April.

If Sara increases her walking time by 5 minutes each week, she will be walking 30 minutes, 4 days a week in her fourth week.

Go for It!

Get a dog that has to go out three times a day. (Is there any other kind?) After lunch I borrow my neighbour's dog and go for a one-hour walk or bike ride every day at the same time. You feel so much better after you have done your activity. Yes, you often have to push yourself to keep in shape, but it's worth it.

— Cato Bayens

Notes: We hope Sara finds a walking partner, a volleyball group, and becomes better informed of what is available in her own community. You see, it's not that hard to meet the minimum requirements!

A minimum of 30 minutes of moderate activity 4 days a week will benefit your health.

Congratulations

You have written a goal statement indicating the level of activity you intend to engage in and when that will happen. You have also spelled out the steps you have to take to ensure that you can meet your goal.

QUICK SUMMARY

- Aim for a balanced lifestyle. Being physically and mentally active will pave the way for balance in the six lifetime goal categories.

- Setting goals will help you identify and clarify your physical activity goals as well as other personal goals. Use the four goal-setting guidelines to set your goals.

- Remember the steps. It's the steps that turn your goal into a reality.

In this chapter:

- Find out why they walk, hike, and canoe for their health and enjoyment.

- Read what our contributors have to say about the activities they love so well: cross-country skiing, curling, bowling, cycling, and slo-pitch softball.

- Learn about the Senior Games and who to contact across Canada to get involved.

- Numerous Web sites tell you where to find information in your own area.

Man does not cease to play because he grows old, man grows old because he ceases to play.

— George Bernard Shaw (1856–1950),
British playwright

Show Me the Way

Olga and I were on our way to meet up with a group for a day hike when we got into a conversation with a lady in the parking garage. When she asked about our day packs, we told her we were going on a hike. She immediately said, "Just the other day, my husband mentioned he would like to go for a hike but he doesn't know where to go. Where do you folks go?" We responded as best we could in the few moments we had to spare and continued on our way.

In hindsight I realize that I should have pulled out a city map, spread it across the trunk of my car and said:

Look at all the green coloured areas on this map. Green signifies parks, and there are hundreds of them. Most parks have walking trails that extend for miles, more than you can cover in a day. Tell your husband that if he wants to go for a hike in the city, get a map, pick any green space and go! He'll be able to walk for months and never cover the same ground twice. If he wants go for a hike outside the city, he should check out the library, the Internet, and the book stores.

There must be thousands of people out there who simply don't know how or where to go for walk or a hike. They may be new to the area or they may have lived their entire adult lives without being aware of the walking and cycling paths in the beautiful parks just a few blocks from where they live.

Activities Close-Up

This chapter will tell you where to look for information about your favourite activity in every province and territory. You will find in-depth looks at such activities as walking, hiking, canoeing, cross-country skiing, cycling, and Seniors Games across Canada. If you are in doubt about what activity you want to get involved in, this chapter should resolve your concerns.

If you have been inactive for some time, there is no magic wand that will turn you into a fit and healthy individual. You have to get up and go often enough to benefit your health. Edward Stanley (1917–1994) had this to say about exercise:

> *"Those who think they have not time for bodily exercise will sooner or later have to find time for illness."*

Walking

Walking ranks number one on the list of most popular physical activities in Canada. According to a 1998 survey of Canadian adults by the

Canadian Fitness and Lifestyle Research Institute, most people chose to walk as a physical activity but they don't walk briskly enough or far enough to achieve any health benefit. Hopefully, this book will help change that. The message for these folks is to keep on walking, just pick up the pace and add a little distance.

Walk for Your Health

When I was a boy, my dad kept at me with one or more of these admonitions:

- Stand up straight
- Pull your shoulders back
- Walk smartly
- Pick up your feet

 Go for It!

People usually have good intentions about exercising, but after a short time they find excuses and stop. Get a few people together and set aside a day or two each week to do something active. Take turns with the organization and planning and get everyone involved.

— Renate Juelich

They say that walking is something you can do without any lessons, but when I see some folks amble along I think they could benefit from my Dad's counsel. I recently observed two women doing a "mall walk." Presumably they were there for the express purpose of benefiting their health, yet one woman had both hands in her pockets as she strolled along and her partner had both hands clasped behind her back. To derive a health benefit they should have picked up their pace and let their arms swing naturally from the shoulder. Try it and watch what happens: with each step your right arm swings forward as your left leg moves forward and vise versa. Also notice that as you walk faster, the speed of your arm swing also increases. So, as you walk, allow your arms to swing naturally and let your hands, arms, and shoulders relax.

With walking, you can set your own schedule and you can do it anytime. You can walk alone, with a partner, or with a group. Best of all, it doesn't cost anything and it's virtually injury-free.

Most people walk because they know it's beneficial to their health. Years ago when I and thousands like me walked and walked around the track at the Toronto Rehab Centre after heart surgery you can be sure that we knew exactly why we were there and it wasn't for a "walk in the park." It was to improve our cardiovascular fitness. Walking is an aerobic exercise that gets the heart beating faster so that it transports oxygen-rich blood from the lungs to the muscles. Walking is at the core of rehab treatment for many ailments, not just heart problems.

Walking briskly is just as beneficial for your overall health as running, but without the negative side effects. Studies show that walking briskly on a regular basis can reduce blood pressure, increase the efficiency of your heart and lungs, and burn excess calories. It can be a valuable part of a weight-loss program as well as a tonic for your mind. I have had a lower back problem for most of my adult life, and I find that walking is one of the best ways for me to avoid the onset of back pain. I can personally vouch for the fact that a brisk walking routine makes me feel better, sleep better, and improves my outlook on life. Try it and I'll bet you'll feel the same way.

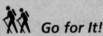 **Go for It!**

Retirement isn't about getting old, it is about opportunity. For the first time in your life, you are in control and free to do the things you always wanted to do. You can learn new skills, participate in clubs, organizations, interest groups, and travel. The fitter you are the more you will enjoy. If you start making positive changes early in your life it will be easier to stay fit and active in retirement.

— Louise Tye

Walk Anywhere

You can walk just about anywhere you please. When you step out your door you can walk the sidewalks in your area, along river trails, on bike trails, nature trails, and public parks. You can join a group of mall-walkers and do your walking indoors during the winter months before the stores open. Olga and I often walk in a nearby shopping mall during the winter months. Whenever you do a mall walk, find a set of steps and briskly walk up and down the steps a few times. It's a great way to build up your leg muscles.

As with any exercise, take it easy at the beginning and build up your pace and distance as your stamina improves. Don't just stroll or shuffle along, hold your head up and walk smartly. Wear good quality comfortable running/walking shoes that provide good support and don't cause blisters. Always bring along a bottle of water and drink it liberally, especially in hot weather. There are some neat devices on the market that fit onto your belt for carrying your bottle of water.

Your Walking Speed

It's a good idea to know your walking speed. There are several ways to do that. In an area of your choice, drive your car for a distance of let's say three kilometres. Later, walk that exact same route and record how many minutes it took. Now you can calculate your walking speed in minutes per kilometres or minutes per mile. One mile in 15 minutes is a very fast walk, and if you walk a mile in 20 minutes you're no slouch for it's still a brisk pace. How do you know how fast you should walk? One easy way is to do what's called the "talk test": if you can't catch your breath or if you are unable to carry on a conversation with your partner you are walking too fast or too strenuously. Always pay attention to how you feel both during your walk and the next day. You can also check with your doctor or another health professional.

If you are presently physically inactive, we urge you to give walking a try. Begin with shorter walks of 10 to 15 minutes, 3 or 4 times a week. Gradually, over time, increase your pace and distance. Once you reach 2 miles in 30 or 40 minutes you've got it made.

Enjoy It

Walking will be more enjoyable if you walk with your spouse, a friend, or a group. If possible find a pleasant park for your walk instead of pounding the pavement. If you find yourself getting bored with your walks, try a different route or an entirely different location. Participate in community walkathons for charity and consider joining a walking group. It's fun and you will feel better for it.

Why Do I Walk?
by Ed Cunningham

Why do I walk? 'Tain't no mystery —
Wanna have a good medical history.
Doctor told me walkin' is great —
Helps them blood cells circulate.
Great for the lungs, great for the ticker,
Can't nothin' getcha in better shape quicker.
Feels so healthy, feels so sweet,
Pumpin' my arms and flappin' my feet,
Moldin' my muscles, firmin' my form,
Pantin' like a pack mule, sweatin' up a storm.
Keeps me youthful, keeps me loose,
Tightens my tummy and shrinks my caboose.
Beats bein' lazy —
Why do I walk? Maybe I'm crazy!

Hiking

Although walking and hiking have their similarities, hiking is sufficiently different to deserve a heading of its own. Hiking is more strenuous than walking, hiking trails are usually over rough and hilly terrain, and it's a given that you wear hiking boots on every hike. A hike is normally a full day outing, and you don't usually find a hiking trail at the end of your driveway.

When I think of hiking I immediately recall my hikes on the Bruce Trail in Ontario, and, more recently, my hikes with the Seniors For Nature Canoe Club (SFNCC). For those who may be thinking of joining an outdoor club, let me briefly describe hiking with the SFNCC, a club we have belonged to for the past 13 years.

Activities at the SFNC include canoeing, camping, hiking, cross-country skiing, and cycling. Some members participate in all these activities while others like us find that two or three activities are sufficient. In a typical year the club program will include about 90 outings in a variety of activities, all led by club members.

Our hikes take place every Tuesday during the fall, winter, and early spring. Everyone planning to participate in a day hike arrives at the scheduled meeting place shortly before 10:00 a.m. Depending on the weather and location, attendance will vary from 10 to 30 hikers. There is a lot of milling about as people greet one another with hugs and hand shakes. Soon we are all busy lacing up our hiking boots, readying our day packs and gear for the hike. Instinctively, everyone ensures that his or her bottle of water is in place, for hiking and drinking water go hand in hand.

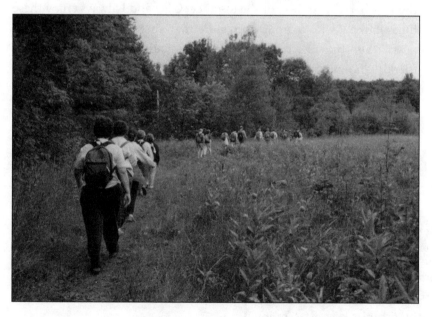

Club members on a hike.

Near the appointed time of 10:00 a.m. the leader calls everyone together for a short briefing. He or she advises about practical things like the type of terrain, the distance of the hike, where we will stop for lunch, and the locations of drop-out points for those who may not want to go the full distance. Sometimes the hikers are familiar with the trail, sometimes not. The leader will have scouted the trail beforehand to check on distance, terrain, and general difficulty of the hike. Hikes take place on trails within the Greater Toronto Area or within an hour's drive of the city.

Hikes will vary in distance from 10 to 15 kilometres. Everyone wears hiking boots as the trails are often rocky. The trails are almost always hilly, and depending on the time of the year the surface may be wet. Hikers are cautioned not to go ahead of the leader and to stay ahead of the sweep. (The sweep is the person designated to bring up the rear and make sure no one is left behind.)

We stop somewhere along the trail for lunch about noon and usually get back to our starting place between two and three o'clock in the afternoon, ready for the drive home. Everyone thanks the leader for the outing, there are more goodbyes, and we all head home. Regardless of the weather, the terrain, or the distance, Olga and I always enjoy these hikes. Hiking with a group does more than improve your physical fitness; it also provides a pleasant time for sharing and socializing with friends who vary in age from 55 to over 80. We arrive home feeling tired but fit and always thankful that we are physically able to enjoy the great outdoors and the company of friends.

If you are interested in hiking, get together with a friend or family member and give it a try. If you like it, consider joining a hiking group in your area. Make the usual inquiries and you will find several groups to choose from. Try to find a group that caters to your age group and hikes in areas within an hour's drive of where you live. Your only major expenditure will be a pair of good hiking boots.

Hiking Trails Everywhere

If you have ever wondered where to look for hiking trails, your search is over. In the pages that follow you will be able to find every major trail in the

 Go for It!

Health concerns, flexibility of the joints and muscles play a role, as does the promise of better memory through physical activity. But the overriding motivation for me is that I do what I enjoy, and am grateful that I can still do it, with friends whom I cherish.

— Margaret Ghattas

100

country. First we list numerous Web sites that will provide you with detailed information about trails, then we give you phone numbers to call for written information about hiking trails by province and territory.

If you take up hiking as an outdoor activity, you'll have lots of company. The famous Bruce Trail in Ontario, for instance, has a membership of 7,500. Regardless of your location in Canada, there is an abundance of trails to choose from, so get your hiking boots ready for a trek to some new and interesting places.

There are three basic sources of trail information:

- word of mouth from other hikers,
- printed material from book stores, libraries, and trail associations, and
- the Internet.

On the Internet

It is beyond the scope of this book to list every hiking trail in Canada, so we settled on a more efficient method. Below, we provide you with a dozen or more Web site addresses that will lead you to the trails you want to find. First we list Web sites that provide trail information for all of Canada, and then we list sites that apply to specific provinces. For even more hiking information, check out our Web site at www.after50.ca.

If you don't have Internet access at home, check with your local library. Many libraries offer free Internet access.

The Trans Canada Trail

The Trans Canada Trail will eventually wind its way through every province and territory. At 16,000 kilometres, it will be longest trail of its kind in the world. The trail will accommodate walking, cycling, horseback riding, cross-country skiing, and, where appropriate, snowmobiling. Approximately 75 percent of the trail will be built on existing trails, abandoned railway lines, and Crown lands, with the remaining 25 percent being new trails. At the time of writing, more than 50 percent of the trail has been completed, and it is expected to be "substantially complete" by the fall of 2005. A series of Trans Canada Trail guidebooks are planned for publication in the very near future.

For links to Trans Canada Trail information for provinces and territories visit its Web site at www.tctrail.ca, or e-mail: info@tctrail.ca. Phone toll free: 1-800-465-3636.

Out-There

Out-There may be Canada's largest outdoor Web site. It provides a wealth of useful information to an enthusiastic and growing outdoor market. The site includes information about travel, nature appreciation, and ecotourism, along with the new generation adventure sports. It will link you to every significant hiking trail in Canada, provincial parks, bird sanctuaries, adventure books, and most every other sort of outdoor interest you may have, from hiking to dog-sledding. Check it out at www.out-there.com.

TrailPAQ

Trailpaq.com is a one-stop Web site destination for trail information across Canada. It includes information about heritage trails, hiking trails, national trails, and local trails in every province. TrailPAQ also provides considerable detail for each trail, such as trail location, distance, type of surface, parking, and washroom information. Compaq (the computer company) states that more than 1,000 trails have been entered into its TrailPAQ database and additional trails are being added daily. This is an amazing site from which you can click your way to hundreds of sites from one end of Canada to the other. It's a new venture, but it is growing by leaps and bounds. Check it out at www.trailpaq.com.

American Trails

This is a comprehensive site with links to numerous trails and related topics across Canada and the U.S. The address is www.americantrails.org.

Trailmonkey: Hiking & Backpacking

This site provides maps and trails coverage for the world. Click on Canada and you will be presented with a vast array of choices in your search for an exciting hike. The address is www.trailmonkey.com/hikingtr.htm.

Trails by Province

Out-There, a Web site we referred to earlier, has a tremendous quantity of data that is easy to access and nicely organized by province. Again, visit the site at www.out-there.com. Here are some others:

Alberta

Trailmonkey provides interesting information on trails and maps not only for Alberta but also the North-West Territories, Yukon, and British Columbia. Go to: www.trailmonkey.com/canadahike.htm.

British Columbia

Boreas Backcountry Adventures provides comprehensive coverage of hiking throughout B.C. You will find treks, descriptions, beautiful pictures, and plenty of surprises as you explore this site, found at www.boreasbackcountry.com.

Newfoundland

Newfoundland's East Coast Trail is a 310-kilometre route mainly south of St. John's. On this trail you will see beautiful scenery, tiny fishing villages, giant icebergs, and whales in the sea. Learn more about it at www.eastcoasttrail.com.

Nova Scotia

Entitled Nature's Resorts, this site provided by the Nova Scotia Parks Department is not only comprehensive but interestingly prepared with maps, charts, and pictures. Take a look: http://parks.gov.ns.ca/dayuse/trails.html.

Ontario

Here's an interesting site with loads of links from Hike Ontario: www.hikeontario.com.

The Bruce Trail is the oldest marked hiking trail in Canada. It is 800 kilometres in length, with another 200 kilometres of side trails along the Niagara Escarpment between Niagara Falls and Tobermory. The Bruce Trail Association Web site is at www.brucetrail.org.

Prince Edward Island

P.E.I. has a well-organized site for presenting trail information. Begin with the InfoPEI site, www.gov.pe.ca/infopei, then click your way to Community Trails, the Confederation Trail, and finally Demonstration Woodlots (the Forest Management Woodlots). You will find every trail in the province along with such details as trail length and points of interest along the trail.

Quebec

This "Go Take a Hike" web site offers a wide range of hiking information for Quebec as well as several areas of the United States. Visit: http://pages.citenet.net/users/ctmx1141.

Yukon and N.W.T

Here's a great site from Out-There for the Canol Heritage Trail and other sites in the North-West Territories and the Yukon. Go to: www.out-there.com/hkg_nt.htm and www.normanwells.com/attract.

Check out the Web sites, find a trail that's right for you, and take a hike. We hope you enjoy your outing and go back for more.

Trail User's Code

Before you set foot on the trails take a few moments to read through the following Trail User's Code, which has been reproduced from the "Bruce Trail Guidebook." Everyone who walks a trail should be familiar with this guide and abide by the code. Please remember that trails are maintained by volunteers and it is volunteers who have to carry out the litter many people leave behind.

Trail User's Code

Hike only along marked routes.
Do not climb fences — use the stiles (steps for crossing over a fence).
Respect the privacy of people living along the trail.
Leave the trail cleaner than you found it — carry out all litter.
Light cooking fires at official campsites only.
Leave flowers and plants for others to enjoy.
Do not damage live trees or strip off bark.
Keep dogs on a leash, especially on or near farmland.
Protect and do not disturb wildlife.
Leave only your thanks and take nothing but photographs.

How to Order Printed Materials by Province

You can obtain written materials on hiking, cycling, and skiing trails, as well as canoe routes and much more by ordering the "Parks" booklet from your provincial tourism office.

Canoeing

If you want to add canoeing to your list of activities check the phone book for a listing of the canoe clubs in your area. To give you an idea of what you may find in a canoe club, here is an overview of the Seniors For Nature Canoe Club activities.

As with most sports, you must learn how to do it. Learning how to stern (steer) a canoe requires both instruction and practise. A prerequisite for membership in some clubs is that you know how to swim and stern a canoe. Fortunately, canoeing classes are not difficult to find. Check the phone book and sporting goods stores to find a flat-water canoeing school in your area.

Our club paddles on flat-water lakes and rivers from May to September. We have one-day canoe outings every Tuesday and a variety of multi-day car camping and wilderness outings throughout the season. Although most members own their own canoe, the club owns several canoes that members may borrow for club outings at any time. As with hiking, all canoe outings are planned, organized, and led by the club members.

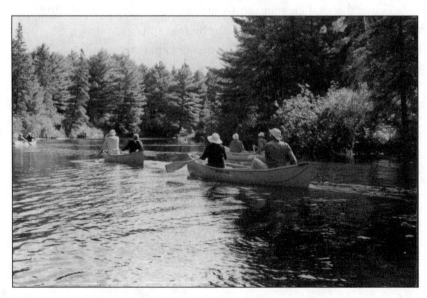

Club members on a canoe outing.

Whatever activity you are involved in, there always seems to be a lot preparation required to get organized and to get where you want to go. Canoeing is no exception, and I have come to realize that it's all part of the enjoyment. One of the first tasks is to get your canoe onto the roof of your car. Just getting it up there and strapped down requires a degree of muscle work, stretching, and know-how by the two people involved.

If it's a day outing, we start canoeing at 10:00 a.m. and continue until noon when we stop for a lunch. After lunch we usually get in another couple hours of paddling before heading back to shore. Then we pack up, tie down the canoes, and head for home. On a wilderness or car camping trip, we would cook outdoors, sleep in a tent, and paddle for two or three days in a row. Under normal weather conditions flat-water canoeing is a pleasant, low-impact aerobic activity, and there is always time to enjoy the sights and sounds of the great outdoors.

Throughout the whole exercise of paddling and handling the gear, everyone is expected to pull his or her own weight. If you are paddling on a lake and a strong wind comes up, you may be put to the test, for there's no alternative but to give it all you've got and paddle as fast and as hard as you can to make it to your destination.

You may be thinking, "That's a lot of effort for a few hours of canoeing," and you might be right. But consider the benefits to your health and well-being:

- Every time you reach forward for another stroke of the paddle you give yourself a good stretch. Every time you pull the paddle back through the water you strengthen the muscles in your arms, stomach, back, and hands.
- You burn off a heap of calories.
- With all that paddling you add to the health of your heart.
- You have fun and enjoy your day as you socialize with a group of wonderful people with similar interests.
- You sleep more soundly that night and feel more rested the next morning.

And besides, canoeing provides an opportunity to enjoy nature at its best. You may spot a blue heron swoop up from its perch and fly overhead. You'll enjoy the peacefulness of it all, the sound of the birds as they chirp and flit from tree to tree. You may hear the splash as a beaver's tail hits the water. And you will certainly chuckle as you hear Rudi's latest tall tale. Wow! Let's do it again next week.

Cross-County Skiing
by Gerda Tismer

The word is out: the 60 to 80-plus year olds are fit! The staff in the ski shop, most of them 50 or more years my junior, no longer patronize me. No longer are the members of my age group viewed as oddities on the cross-country ski trails. In fact, on weekdays the seniors dominate the ski areas. My husband Rudi and I try to get out cross-country skiing at least twice a week during the winter months.

Most of my skiing over the past 25 years has been done on groomed, mostly track set trails at various resorts and provincial parks.

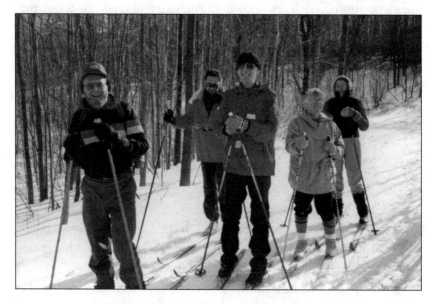

Club members cross-country skiing.

Usually, Rudi and I stride out together for a warm-up and then go our separate ways. Having always belonged to a ski club, I meet old and current acquaintances along the way, and we stay together for a while. I manage 18 to 25 kilometres between mid-morning and four in the afternoon, which among regular skiers is nothing to write home about, but the point is, you do your best without wearing yourself out.

From my experience, cross-country skiing is a valuable cardiovascular exercise for people of all ages, one that does not make great demands on the joints. There are three components that work on your body: the climbing, which demands deep breathing; the controlled downhill glide, which gives you the satisfaction of being master over your skis; and the rhythmic, diagonal stride which involves the whole body in a coordinated, almost flowing motion.

One of the most interesting places to ski in Ontario is Wasaga Beach Provincial Park at the southern end of Georgian Bay. Why would skiing along a beach be particularly interesting? Well, the park is actually a dune landscape away from the water. One of the trails winds gently up a gully to the top of an impressive high dune, then goes along a horseshoe-shaped ridge with fabulous vistas before dropping down in stages. But pleasant scenery can be found at all our southern Ontario ski areas. Most have comfortable, if sometimes crowded, cafeterias. Some offer the romantic atmosphere of a hut way out on the trails where you can light a fire, have your lunch, and use an authentic outhouse. Brrr!

For winter vacations we have often headed to Mont Ste. Anne or the Mont Tremblant area in "La Belle Province." Skiing the extensive trail system on day excursions that took us many miles from home base called for a degree of self-reliance. The question was always there — "Are we well enough prepared for weather changes, a minor accident, or an equipment breakdown?"

Besides meeting a lot of like-minded people, joining a club offers other advantages: relaxing on a chartered bus instead of gripping the steering wheel, especially on snowy roads, ski lessons by certified instructors, and reduced trail fees. If you feel like the new kid on the block, ski lessons are an easy way to "settle in."

All through the sixties, the two of us, along with friends, extended our backcountry skiing to snow camping once a year. I can still see myself flying down a slope slightly out of control, a sooty pot in one hand, fighting the backward pull of a big pack. The pack won out. On another occasion we pulled a sled loaded with gear to a suitable tenting spot miles away from the highway. The sled overturned several times. There is nothing like wiggling into a cold sleeping bag in a cold tent, wearing all the clothes you wore during the day plus some more. That experience could only be matched by waking up to frozen vapor from our breathing on the sleeping bags and tent walls and climbing into half-frozen boots. Why did we do it? Because of the starry nights, the crackling campfires, the camaraderie, the banter, the laughter when the foil-wrapped sausages turned to charcoal in the hot ashes. If cross-country skiing is preventive medicine, I find it easy to swallow.

Curling
by Bruce Deachman, for the Canadian Curling Association

I've been covering curling as a journalist for the *Ottawa Citizen* for five years now, from its elite performers to the once-a-year neophytes. I've meandered hundreds of years into the sport's past, poking into its nooks and crannies, and I've followed its most recent developments.

I know these numbers as well as I know my own address: More than a million Canadians curl at least once every year at one of the country's 1,200 clubs. About three-quarters of a million did it on at least a monthly basis this past year, and most curl on a fairly non-competitive basis. In terms of demographics, according to the Print Measurement Bureau's most recent figures, curlers tend to be slightly above-average in areas traditionally associated with success; more white-collar workers than in the country in general, with a higher education and higher earnings than the national average.

Yet, despite the relative professional success of its participants, curling is the sport with perhaps the greatest grassroots base. As Jean Sonmor wrote in her book, *Burned by the Rock*, "These Canadians are farmers, fishermen, stockbrokers. They run computers, hairdressing salons, or supermarkets. The mix is as diverse as the country."

There are as many reasons to curl as there are curlers. Compared to sports like golf, hockey, or skiing, curling is affordable: a typical curling membership runs anywhere from $100 to $300 per year, while the cost of equipment is hardly daunting when stacked beside just about any other activity. The entry-level skills required are minimal, too. Curling clubs openly welcome curlers of all ages and abilities. You're never too young, or too old, to start curling.

With 1,200 clubs in Canada, you're never too far from one, either, whether you live downtown in a sprawling metropolis or in the shadow of a lone grain elevator.

It terms of curling's fitness and cardiovascular benefits, it's is an excellent sport for all ages, with the output of energy, especially when sweeping teammates' rocks, fairly self-regulated. In other words, you can get a good workout when you want one, but you can also avoid undue stress when necessary.

But none of this, not the reasonable cost, the accessibility, or the health benefits, accounts for why most people curl. It certainly doesn't begin to explain why I took it up myself at the beginning of last season after watching from the sidelines for years. Curling, at its heart, is a social sport. Not only do you have three teammates cheering you on, but every team you play against is part of curling's fraternity. You shake hands before the game and again afterwards, joining one another for a post-game soda and social. With every game played, your contact with the world expands, as the six degrees of separation become five, then four, three, two, one, and, finally, non-existent.

Rural curlers already know this. In many communities, the curling club was the third public structure built, just after the church and school. Curling, in smaller, rural populations, is the very thread that ties the community together through long, cold winters.

In cities, curling provides meaningful human contact after a day of avoiding conversation in elevators and eye contact in traffic. It offers an opportunity to be a part of the community again, while enjoying the benefits of competition.

No matter where you participate, though, curling grabs hold of you by its very grassroots and pulls you to the sport's heart, to where the people are, to where you can feel what it's like just to be. It connects us all to one another. As Sonmor put it, "In curling rinks you see viva-cious stay-at-home grandmothers in intense conversation with slick male accountants. On the street, they inhabit different worlds, but here, in the club, they are buddies."

Cycling
by Dave McDonald

The 300 kilometres of cycling paths around the city of Ottawa and over into the Quebec side must be among the best in Canada. I'm just finishing my fourth cycling season here and I'm hooked. For the sum-mer months, I can think of nothing better than a good bike ride to get me outdoors and keep me fit.

Back in April 1999, I was out of shape. Although I have been an avid squash player for 25 years, I got lazy, only played once a week and put on 20 extra pounds. I had just turned 50 and I didn't like the way I felt or the way I looked. Trying to lose weight through jogging or more squash didn't interest me, as they are both hard on the body. I wanted to try something different.

I decided to try cycling as a way to get back into shape and it worked. The price of a "hybrid" style bike was nominal at $450, with another $200 for helmet, gloves, and accessories. I knew that cycling was a wise choice for fitness, but I underestimated the enjoyment I would get from the Ottawa cycling trails.

One of the first things I noticed about cycling was how convenient it was to get on the bike and go for a good ride. I'm lucky, as I can get onto several bike trails within a 15-minute cycle from my house. I recall my initial few efforts on the bike, when my legs and butt were always sore even after a short 30-minute ride. Then the rides started getting longer, easier, and more enjoyable. That first year I was on my bike about 100 times, averaging 20 kilometres a trip. I ride at about 20 kilometres per hour, so the average outing was about 60 minutes. On several occasions, I cycled to the other end of Ottawa or over the bridge into Quebec.

I loved the quiet, demanding rides and the great feeling it gave me when I finished. It gave me a good workout and the physical benefits were apparent. I lost 20 pounds over a 4-month period and I knew that I had found a sport for life.

During my second year of cycling I rode more frequently but for shorter times of between 30 to 60 minutes. I didn't get the intense workout that I did in my first year, but I enjoyed the relaxation and the scenery.

As my fourth season comes to a close I am no longer a novice. This has been my best cycling year — my technique has improved and the longer rides feel easier. It's now September and I have reached my goal of 3,000 kilometres without too much difficulty. My best efforts were a few 100-kilometre trips and some extremely hard outings into the Gatineau Hills.

If you are in the 50-plus category, overweight and out of shape, cycling may be your answer to improved fitness. Cycling is rated as one of the best physical activities for weight loss and fitness improvement provided the rides are long enough and strenuous enough. If you take up cycling as a regular form of exercise, start off slowly with shorter, more leisurely rides and gradually increase both your speed and distance. You may also want to check with your doctor before taking on the more strenuous rides.

A 30- to 45-minute workout 4 times a week will improve your endurance level, strengthen your body, and help you lose weight. You can tell when you are working hard, because that's when your legs pump harder, you breathe harder, and you sweat more. If you hope to achieve a weight loss of 20 to 50 pounds, think of it as a 2- to 3-year project, cycling in the summer and keeping fit with various other activities during the winter months.

Over the years I have acquired a few insights into the area of physical fitness and I would like to pass them on here. Your experiences may be similar.

- More than half the time I don't "feel like" starting the activity. I usually have to psych myself to get my bike out the door or get my squash gear ready and drive to the club.
- After starting the activity, the hardest part is the initial 15 minutes while my body warms up, then it gets easier.

- The best part is after you're warmed up and you are able to unconsciously carry on the activity without focusing on it, while obtaining a euphoric sensation that comes with a good workout.
- I always, always feel good when I am finished. I feel fulfilled knowing that I have physically accomplished something.
- When keeping fit through activities and sports, my body is usually a bit stiff and sore in the mornings. That's okay provided there is no injury and it goes away with activity during the day.
- Pace yourself and learn to trust the way your body feels. Take one or two days off each week and a longer break if you are overly tired or have had enough for a while.

Note:

- There are numerous maps and books available showing cycling trails in all provinces and cities across Canada. They are available at most bicycle retailers.
- If you would like to join a cycling group rather than cycling on your own, check with the parks and recreation department at your city hall; staff there will be able to direct you to the appropriate contact person.

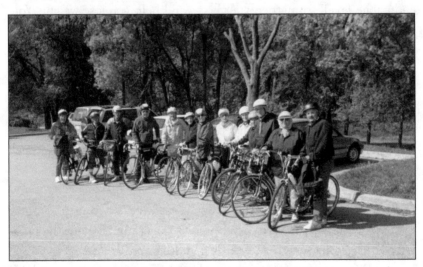

Club members out for a ride.

Bowling

Part of the following is an edited excerpt from the Bowling Proprietors Association of Canada Web site, which can be found at www.bpac.ca.

Bowling is much more than a great sport. It's a favourite pastime world-wide. Bowling is a recreation, a vehicle for family entertainment, a learning ground for the young, and a means of moderate exercise for the aged. Virtually everyone has bowled at some time or another, and millions of Canadians continue to bowl on a regular basis. They also have fun!

In 1972, a program now known as Club 55+ was developed for Canadian senior citizens with the following aims and objectives:

- to encourage seniors to take part in a healthy, lifetime activity,
- to provide a means of moderate exercise on a regular basis, and
- to offer an environment where seniors could socialize with their peers and share in a fun and challenging sport.

More than 20,000 Canadian men and women over the age of 55 take part regularly in a Club 55+ league, where they have an opportunity to socialize with their peers and enjoy some moderate exercise.

Joining a Club 55+ league gives you an opportunity to meet a great many people with similar interests and experiences, and it's a great way to keep active and fit. So drop in to one of your local bowling centres and let them know you'd like to sign up with the program. That's the hard part. The rest is easy — just enjoy yourself!

In his book *Canada Firsts*, Ralph Nader reminds us that Tommy Ryan (1872–1961), a native of Guelph, Ontario literally invented five-pin bowling. About 1909, he reduced the 10 pins down to 5, shaved down the pins on a lathe, used a smaller ball, changed the scoring system, and made it obligatory for a player to knock down the left corner pin before any points could be awarded. The game was an immediate success and soon became one of the most popular sports in Canada and the northern United States.

Senior Games

Senior Games is a recreational program for adults 55 years of age and over. As they say in British Columbia: Sport knows no age barriers when the young at heart take to the field, the pool, and the court.

It's all about fun, fitness, and friends. Senior Games offer people from all walks of life a variety of ways to stay active and involved. Senior Games are held every second year in every province except Nova Scotia, Newfoundland, and Quebec. Some provinces hold both winter and summer games.

Within each province, participants must first qualify at a local community level, then the district level, and finally the provincial level. Winners from the provincial competitions travel to the biennially held Canada Senior Games. When you consider that the Senior Games are held at various provincial levels before reaching the national level, you realize that there truly is a lot of participation. Ontario, for instance, indicates that some 20,000 seniors are involved in its Senior Games.

Typical events at the provincial summer games are shown in the table below.

Typical events at Senior Summer Games	
Bowling (5- and 10-pin)	Golf
Carpet & Lawn bowling	Horseshoes
Cribbage	Slo-pitch softball
Contract bridge	Snooker
Darts	Swimming
Euchre	Tennis
Floor shuffleboard	Walking (prediction)

Other sports included in some provinces:

Badminton, Bocce ball, Curling, Cycling,
Table tennis, Square dancing, Volleyball, and more.

A prediction walk is not a walk against time or against the other participants, but rather it is a contest to see who can come closest to predicting how long it will take to walk a specified distance of three kilometres. These walks are measured to the hundredth of a second and are considered among the best events in the games. It also calls for considerable preparation before the games, as each participant has to do a lot practice walking against a stop watch to get his or her time down to the second.

At present the winter games include the following sanctioned events:

- Alpine skiing
- Badminton
- Curling
- Bowling (5- and 10-pin)
- Hockey
- Prediction Nordic skiing
- Prediction skating

Canada Senior Games

The first ever Canada Senior Games was held from September 11 to 15, 1996, in Regina, Saskatchewan. In attendance were 500 participants from 6 provinces. Events included contract bridge, cribbage, darts, five-pin bowling, golf, horseshoes, lawn bowling, shuffleboard, snooker, swimming, tennis, track, and novice cycling.

As stated in the 1996 Official Souvenir Program from Regina:

> The purpose of the Games is to promote participation by all seniors in an active and enjoyable lifestyle, thus the Canada Senior Games are a means to an end, the promotion of activities for all seniors. Each event at the Canada Senior Games is composed of some combination of Physical Activity, Socialization and/or Mental Stimulation. The key principles are participation and fun.

Join the Fun

If you have not been involved in the Senior Games in your local area why not get involved? Enjoy the fun and the challenge of friendly competition. There are three ways to get involved:

- Be a participant in the events,
- Act as a games official making use of your sports expertise, or
- Be an event organizer or committee member.

Senior Games Contacts

An up-to-date list of Senior Games contacts as well as details of recent and upcoming games in each province and territory will be maintained on our Web site, www.after50.ca. To keep the list current, we ask that members of the Senior Games associations of each province or territory submit changes in information via e-mail to jim.olga@after50.ca.

QUICK SUMMARY

- You now have first-hand accounts of the pleasure and fulfillment people derive from taking a brisk walk, hiking, canoeing, cross-country skiing, bowling, curling, and cycling. We hope they will encourage you to participate.

- Thousands of people are actively involved in the Senior Games and they are looking for more. Why not join in the fun? There's a contact person in your area ready to help you get involved.

PART TWO: ACTIVE MIND

In the year 1801 Wilhelm von Humboldt, a German scholar, philosopher, and educator, had this to say:

> True enjoyment comes from activity of the mind
> and exercise of the body; the two are ever united.

It's no secret, the two are "ever united," and this book gives equal weight to the needs of both mind and body. In Part One we devoted five chapters to keeping your body fit, and now Part Two takes direct aim at exercising your mind.

Can we tell you exactly what you should do to keep your mind active? Of course not, but we will try to arouse your interest in becoming mentally active and we will undertake to stimulate your desire to do those things that give you a feeling of self-fulfillment. In short, if you feel somewhat lost and frustrated, with no sense of purpose in your life, we will try to point the way to a happier, more fulfilling lifestyle.

Now that you are retired or about to retire, do you know what you would like to do during your so-called retirement years? If you are still struggling with that question you are not alone, but don't be overly concerned — the purpose of the next five chapters is to help you find the light at the end of that tunnel.

In this part we hope to trigger ideas in your mind by providing examples of what has worked for others. In the pages ahead we explore the benefits of volunteering, the world of computers and the Internet, the thrill of genealogy, the journey of learning, and the love of arts and crafts. These are just some of the areas that have brightened the lives of many who may otherwise be living in boredom and loneliness.

Part Two Summary

Each chapter in this part of the book is a stand-alone topic and may be read in any sequence. To help you focus on the chapters that appeal to you most, here is a brief synopsis of each chapter. Read through this summary, then identify those chapters you are most interested in.

What are your areas of interest?	
Place a check mark opposite the topics of greatest interest to you. Each topic has the potential to make your life more interesting and rewarding.	
Chapter 6 — Lend a Helping Hand As the name suggests, this chapter is all about volunteering, almost always a win-win undertaking. Volunteering generates a lot of personal satisfaction, costs nothing, and places you in contact with others who have similar interests. If you have a desire to help others but don't know how to get started, you will find the answers here.	
Chapter 7 — The Computer & You You may feel that the computer has no place in your life, but don't be too quick to write it off. Why not be fair to yourself and consider the pros and cons before making a decision? Getting involved with today's friendly computer has opened a new world of enjoyment, learning, and accomplishment for thousands. This chapter may be just what you have been searching for.	
Chapter 8 — Tracing Your Ancestors Genealogy is a most fascinating pursuit with rewards at every turn. Like eating a box of chocolates, each bite tastes so good that you feel compelled to go back for more. This chapter will show you how to get started, where to search, how to organize your data, and how to assemble it for sharing with your relatives.	
Chapter 9 — The Learning Journey Continuing education and distance education are commonplace terms in numerous 50-plus homes. If you have an enquiring mind and a desire to learn, this chapter will help speed you on your way. Once you reach the finish line you will love that feeling of accomplishment.	
Chapter 10 — The Joy of Creating & Doing We all derive intense satisfaction from creating even the smallest thing. If you have a void in your life you may find what you are looking for within these pages. This chapter goes well beyond crafts and hobbies to include people activities as well. Once you read this chapter you will never again walk the floor or twiddle your thumbs in boredom.	

In this chapter:

- Learn why 6.5 million Canadians find volunteering a rewarding experience.

- Find out the amazing scope of organizations that depend on volunteers. There is bound to be some way you can help out related to your special area of interest.

- Learn all about volunteer opportunities overseas.

"It is one of the beautiful compensations of life that no man can sincerely help another without helping himself."
— Ralph Waldo Emerson (1803–1882),
American poet and essayist

High Praise for Volunteering

In a press release dated October 28, 1999, Dr. Neena Chappell, director of the Centre on Aging at the University of Victoria, made the following statement:

> People who give their time to a volunteer activity, especially if it involves helping others, are happier and healthier in their later years.

Whether engaged in formal or informal volunteering tasks, Chappell also notes that volunteers seem to derive health benefits from volunteering because they feel that they are useful and making a contribution. "Volunteering is a people-to-people business," says Chappell.

"A lot of the benefit comes from being in touch with others and having an impact on their lives."

When I first read the above comments I wondered if I could find a real-life story to support Dr. Chappell's observations. I sent e-mails to just a few agencies asking for volunteer stories, and in no time at all I had what I was looking for. Here are two stories that confirm that volunteers derive health benefits, feel useful, enjoy being involved in a people-to-people business, and notice a positive impact on their lives. Read on, and I'm sure you will agree.

A Win-Win Encounter
Submitted by Bryony Hollick,
Special Projects Coordinator, Volunteer Burnaby, B.C.

Graham Bolwell worked for many years in the heavy metal industry until a series of heart attacks forced him to stop working while he was still in his 50s. Although deeply depressed, he started volunteering at the Second Street Community School in Burnaby, B.C., helping children learn woodworking. To Graham's surprise, his work with the children had a far greater healing effect on him than the most potent antidepressant.

One of the children was Raymond, a quiet and withdrawn native boy who did not participate in school activities or interact with his classmates. One day while working with Raymond, Graham showed him some

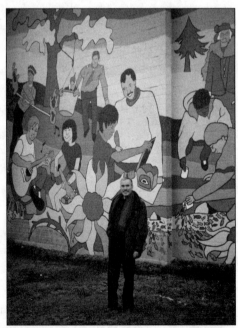

Graham Bolwell in front of the mural depicting himself working with Raymond

122

photos he had taken in the small town of Lilloet, B.C. It so happened that Lilloet was young Raymond's hometown. Suddenly, the quiet, withdrawn boy opened up and began telling stories of his life in Lilloet. He talked about many things, including fishing in his favourite river. Their discussions continued — Raymond was on the mend and so was Graham.

Last year a community mural was designed to celebrate community volunteers. The mural shows Graham helping Raymond make a carved wooden box, and the huge smile on Graham's face confirms his pride in the volunteering experience. The mural is located on the side of the Dolphin Cinema, at 4555 East Hastings St. in Burnaby.

Toques for Preemies
Submitted by Volunteer Nanaimo and Marilyn Guille, Nanaimo, B.C.

A three-pound baby needs all the help it can get to survive. With heat loss being a major obstacle, tiny "toques" for premature babies are in demand in hospital nurseries all over North America.

A Nanaimo woman, Marilyn Guille, started knitting the little caps in her spare time. The demand was so great that she put out a call for more knitters. The response was immediate and overwhelming. Within a few weeks, more women signed up as volunteer knitters, and boxes and bags full of the tiny toques began pouring into the drop-off centre.

As the demand grew, Volunteer Nanaimo got involved, and soon 50 knitters were creating teeny caps and donating them by the boxful to hospitals across the country in towns such as Coquitlam and Victoria in British Columbia; Edmonton and Drayton Valley in Alberta; Barrie, London, and Brampton in Ontario; and upstate New York. Knitters ranged in age from 7 to 92 and most of them turned out one cap a day. In 2002, the Preemie Toque Program hit an all-time high of more than 700 caps delivered in March alone.

The caps keep the tiny babies warm and comfortable during their first struggle in a new environment. New moms worried about their tiny tykes really appreciate this kindness and the homey touch.

Can you help? Of course you can knit caps! If this is a project that tugs at your heartstrings, go to this Web site to find out how to get involved: www.volunteernanaimo.ca/toques.htm.

Everyone Benefits

The National Survey of Giving, Volunteering, and Participating for the year 2000 tells us that 6.5 million volunteers across Canada donated more than 1 billion hours of their time. That's equivalent to more than 549,000 full-time jobs. The report further states that 28 percent of the 55 to 64 age group and 18 percent of the over 65 age group volunteered their time to a charitable or non-profit organization. These numbers clearly indicate that all Canadians, including those over 50, have a right to be proud of the vital role they play in improving the quality of life for so many grateful individuals in their communities.

You Give and You Get Back

As a volunteer, you donate your time and skills to help others for a wide variety of reasons. Yes, volunteering involves a desire to help others, but you should also enjoy what you do and derive personal satisfaction from your volunteer work. Volunteering is a two-way street, an exchange of sorts in which you get something back for your time and skills.

That thought, eloquently expressed by Ralph Waldo Emerson, appears on the cover page of this chapter: It is one of the beautiful com-

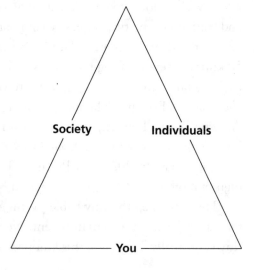

pensations of life that no man can sincerely help another without helping himself.

To ensure that a two-way street exists for the volunteer work you do, you should be selective in the type of volunteer work you choose. Later in this chapter you will find a short questionnaire that will help you decide when and where you want to volunteer.

Benefits of Volunteering

- Volunteering provides personal satisfaction.
- Volunteering provides an opportunity for retired men and women to stay active in their communities.
- Volunteering helps newly retired men and women make the transition from a structured workplace to a lifestyle of choices.
- Studies show that people who volunteer to help others have a higher level of life satisfaction, a stronger will to live, and fewer symptoms of depression and anxiety.

Why People Volunteer

- To help a cause they believe in
- To use and share their skills and experience
- To support a specific organization that has influenced their life
- To help a friend or relative
- Because they feel it's their civic duty
- As a true gift from the heart
- Simply to keep busy
- To learn something new
- Because it gives them a feeling of pride
- To feel good about themselves
- To meet people and make new friends
- To do something quite different from their regular job
- For religious reasons

Finding a Position That Fits

Volunteers offer their gifts of time and talent to a wide range of organizations and an even broader array of activities. Their activities range from serving on the board of directors of a charitable organization to delivering meals to the elderly. Our aim is to make it easy for you to select the organization you are interested in and then be able to contact the right person. For starters, here is a breakdown of eight broad categories of organizations that depend on volunteers to support their work.

1. **Arts and Culture**
   - art galleries and museums
   - zoos and aquariums
   - historical sites
   - festivals

2. **Sports and Recreation Organizations**
   - mostly available within your own community

3. **Social Service Organizations**
   - services for children, youth, and families
   - handicapped people
   - elderly people
   - food banks
   - community services

4. **Health Organizations**
   - hospitals
   - nursing homes
   - mental health and crisis intervention
   - public health and wellness education
   - out-patient health treatment
   - rehabilitative medical services
   - emergency medical services

5. **Religious Organizations**
   - churches
   - mosques
   - synagogues
   - shrines
   - monasteries

6. **Education**
   - literacy
   - ESL
   - libraries
   - schools

7. **The Environment and Parks**
   - federal parks
   - provincial parks
   - conservation areas

8. **International Aid**
   - Canadian Executive Service Organization
   - Canadian Crossroads International
   - CUSO
   - Voluntary Service Overseas

   ... and many others

Actual Volunteer Postings

To provide you with a realistic view of the volunteer opportunities available within some of the categories mentioned above, here are a number of edited excerpts from actual listings of volunteer opportunities. Names of organizations and other details have been removed.

Excerpts from Actual Postings — Social Services

- Drivers to collect perishable food from supermarkets, restaurants, and caterers and deliver it to social service agencies.
- Volunteers to teach exercise classes to senior residents with limited mobility.
- A distress centre is looking for empathetic friendly volunteers to assist on the telephone lines. Answer calls from the lonely, depressed, or even suicidal. For as little as four hours a week you can help ease someone's pain and support them through difficult time.
- A small grassroots organization dedicated to helping all victims of violence is in need of energetic volunteers to serve on its board of directors. Some of the tasks would involve creating and implementing fundraising activities and helping to secure corporate funding.
- Association for the blind needs volunteers to help visually impaired persons: go for walks, read their mail, go shopping, etc.
- Volunteer lawyer needed to assist in legal clinics. You would be responsible for pointing out options that are available to women regarding legal information and referring them to the appropriate sources.

Excerpts from Actual Postings — Health

- Volunteers to assist with a unique swim program for children with multiple disabilities. Help a child prepare for the pool, accompany the child to a therapeutic pool, and get the child ready to leave.
- Support care volunteers are needed to prepare meals, clean houses, and interact with residents who are living with AIDS.
- Daytime volunteers are needed to help disabled riders get their horses ready and lead the horses during a one-hour class. Great opportunity to work with horses and truly wonderful people.

Excerpts from Actual Postings — Education

- Volunteers with excellent English as well as good administrative and computer skills for office work and data entry.
- A literacy organization is seeking board members. Attend and participate in monthly meetings of the board of directors. Vote on various issues and policies. Participate on a committee, e.g. newsletter, program, funding, or personnel.
- Tutor youth in math, English, science, or computers in the evening. Excellent communication and interpersonal skills required.
- Volunteers to work with individuals with a brain injury to teach them how to operate computers and basic software programs.

Volunteers Make the Difference

From the Alzheimer Society to the YMCA/YWCA Canada, the list of organizations in need of volunteers is endless. If you have a special interest in a certain charitable cause or organization, look there first and you may find a volunteer opportunity that suits you perfectly.

Four Ways to Volunteer

Here are four ways to get in touch with the right people. Who you offer to help will depend on which organization you are interested in and the type of volunteer work you are looking for.

1. Contact Your Local Volunteer Centre

Volunteer centres are independent community-based organizations with a primary focus on recruitment and referral of volunteers. The vast majority of volunteering takes place through volunteer centres across Canada. These centres have a large database of volunteer opportunities to fill and a staff of qualified interviewers (volunteers, of course) who guide you through the process of selecting the volunteer position best suited for you. There is no fee and no pressure, just the pleasant experience of searching for and finding that special position that will bring satisfaction to your life.

If you contact a volunteer centre with a request to volunteer for an organization that recruits its own volunteers directly, the volunteer centre will willingly advise you how to get in touch with that organization.

2. Contact the Organization Directly

Organizations such as hospitals, museums, and art galleries usually recruit and administer their own volunteers. If you know the name of the organization you would like to volunteer for, and if they do their own volunteer recruiting, you should contact them directly.

3. Volunteer over the Internet with VOE

Volunteer Canada is the national umbrella organization for the volunteer centres across the country. Volunteer Canada engages in research, training, and other national initiatives designed to increase community participation across the country.

In 1999 Volunteer Canada set up a program called Volunteer Opportunities Exchange (VOE) whereby those with Internet access may complete a volunteer profile, then forward it to Volunteer Canada via the Internet. VOE will then match you with a volunteer position that takes into consideration your location and the type of volunteer work you are looking for. Volunteer Canada's Web site is at www.volunteer.ca. The Volunteer Opportunities Exchange (VOE) can be found at www.volunteer.ca/volunteer/voe.htm. You can also contact Volunteer Canada by phone at 1-800-670-0401 or 613-231-4371, or by e-mail at volunteer.canada@sympatico.ca.

4. Charity Village

Charity Village is identified as Canada's super-site for the non-profit sector. It supports and serves 175,000 registered Canadian charities and non-profit organizations. Some of its site destinations are designed for non-profit managers, staffers, and fundraisers, while others are primarily for volunteers, donors, and supporters.

Charity Village went on-line in 1995 and quickly became an important source of on-line news, jobs, and services for the Canadian non-profit community. Charity Village states that its site includes more than 3,000 pages of information and is accessed more than 7 million times each

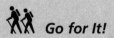 **Go for It!**

Join volunteer groups and aim to become volunteer of the year.
— John Galbraith

month. Whether you are a volunteer offering your skills or an organization seeking help, this amazing site fulfills both needs. Just a couple of clicks and you can find volunteer information for most major centres across Canada. Wherever you live, this site is worth a visit. It can be found at www.charityvillage.com. Charity Village can also be reached by phone at 905-453-7321.

Be a Hospital Volunteer

Volunteers are valuable members of the hospital community. That point was stressed recently by Renta Ivankovic, coordinator of volunteer services, as she spoke to a group of 30 potential volunteers at the Trillium Health Centre in Mississauga. She said, "You are not just a volunteer, you are part of the team." The potential volunteers at the meeting I attended came from all walks of life and all age groups, including seniors.

Volunteers are respected and appreciated by staff and patients alike and they are welcomed in almost every area of hospital services. As a volunteer you may provide direct support to the patients, assist the public, work with hospital staff, or become involved in a fundraising project. Without volunteers, hospitals would be unable to offer the same degree of care to their patients. Hospital volunteers make this possible by offering their time and their skills for the benefit of the patients.

Typical Hospital Procedure

Most hospitals follow a procedure similar to the one outlined below. These steps are necessary for the safety and security of patients, visitors, staff, and volunteers alike.

1. **Attend an information session.** Interested members of the community are invited to attend an information session at the hospital. These sessions are usually booked in advance, so if you wish to attend, contact volunteer services at your hospital and register well ahead of the information session.

2. **Complete an application form.** At the information session, you will be given an application form. Complete it and arrange a date and time for an interview with the appropriate hospital staff member.

3. **Attend a one-on-one interview.** If you have a special interest, such as wanting to work with children, it is at this interview that you can make your preference known. If you are unsure of where you would like to be placed, a staff member will work with you to help arrange the best possible placement.

4. **Provide references.** The volunteer coordinator will check your references following the interview.

5. **Get occupational health testing.** Volunteers must complete a tuberculosis surveillance test and provide evidence of immunity against rubella, measles, and chicken pox prior to beginning a volunteer placement.

6. **Attend an orientation session.** Orientation will help prepare you for your role on the health care team.

7. **Successfully complete service training.** This may include a tour of the key areas, introduction to staff, and a complete review of your service description and duties.

Make a Commitment

The coordinator of volunteer services at a hospital may have the responsibility of juggling the assignments and hours of service for more than 1,000 volunteers. For that reason, most hospitals require that volunteers meet certain standards and make a minimum time commitment. Here's what most hospitals expect from their volunteers:

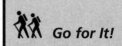 **Go for It!**

I recently read that the more socially connected people are in life, the healthier they tend to be.
— Ken Holden

- a commitment of at least one shift (three or four hours) per week for a period of six months,
- possession of a valid Health Card,
- willingness to sign a volunteer confidentiality agreement, and
- willingness to participate in the orientation session, various training programs, meetings, and continual learning activities.

Typical Hospital Programs

Although the specific tasks will vary from one hospital to another, volunteers have an opportunity to become involved in a wide variety of areas.

Assisting Patients
- Cardiac diagnostics
- Patient care units
- Emergency/Urgent care centre
- Oncology clinic
- Paediatrics
- Meal assistance
- Special outings
- Rehabilitation

- Long-term care
- Psychiatry
- Obstetrics

Assisting Staff
- Office clerical support
- Health records
- Administration

Assisting the Public
- Emergency reception
- Gift shop
- Craft sales
- Information desk
- Hospitality
- Ambulatory clinic
- Pre-Op centres

Community Outreach
- Special projects

Fundraising

What's in It for You?

Long-time volunteers say that after spending a day helping others you realize that you have also helped yourself in some way. That's the main thing, but in addition you may get a thank you for a job well done and you may be mentioned in a newsletter. There is one certainty: in helping others you will have the personal satisfaction of knowing that you made a difference.

From the *Armagh News*

Armagh provides a program of supportive housing for abused women and their children in Mississauga, Ontario. When Olga and I dropped off a box of toys at the beautiful Armagh home just before Christmas, we picked up its current newsletter. As I read through it I spotted a most inspiring item from one of its volunteers. I was so impressed with Jean's letter that I obtained her permission to include it this book. I am certain that her words echo the thoughts of all volunteers wherever they are, and if you are toying with the idea of becoming a volunteer, Jean's letter may help you make up your mind.

A Remarkable Experience
by Jean Donato

When I look back on the beginning of my volunteering at Armagh, I remember a feeling of stage fright, eagerness, and joy. I was sincerely grateful that this remarkable organization was willing to accept me into their service. I was accepted warmly by the staff who made Armagh a comfortable, caring haven.

It has been a remarkable experience. There have been occasions when I was able to interact with some of the residents — a young woman with beautiful, engaging twins came to visit me as I worked in the office. An older lady, shy but friendly, joined me for a little while on several occasions to say hello and to talk. She liked talking to me about her daughter, who was also a resident.

For me, the first and most important factor in volunteering for this service is the rewarding experience of being able to help. The realization that I could contribute. Commitment in volunteering is not to be taken lightly. If one signs on, then that commitment must be followed. My own commitment and reason for volunteering is that I am giving something back to my community.

I am grateful for and blessed in my own personal life. Sharing my time and efforts and sincerity in this volunteer role enhances my well-being as I hope it enhances the well-being of those served.

Out of the Ordinary

Some volunteer opportunities are sufficiently unusual or out of the ordinary that they deserve special mention. Let's look at a few of them.

Would You Like to Be a Docent?
by Mary A. Rochon

We do things for different reasons at various stages of life.

When I was operating my commercial fine art gallery in downtown Toronto, it was a venture for financial gain, as well as a love of art. After almost 10 years of wrestling with marketing and sales it was time to seek out a more self-fulfilling career. Following a period of investigation, the path narrowed and led me to inquiring about being a docent at the Art Gallery of Ontario on Dundas Street in Toronto. And you say, "What is a docent?"

The museum or art gallery docent is neither a teacher nor a curator, an administrator nor a recreation leader, but a combination of all of these and more.

Tour guide, docent, volunteer, interpreter, and instructor are some of the names given to those who "translate," or decode, or explain and describe exhibits. These names identify volunteer educators who meet with the public and provide information to them about exhibits. The effective educator, however, discloses more than simply exhibit information. Tour effectiveness is a product of the guide's organization, preparation, and choice of tour strategy, as well as personal style, knowledge, and enthusiasm.

Tour guides in museums today are, for the most part, creative, imaginative, intelligent people who can incite enthusiasm in visitors and offer new insights about our society. They are in fact para-professionals. In no other field are volunteers doing such responsible work. They are absolutely essential to museums as guides who interpret exhibits for visitors. They can learn and enrich their own lives along the way.

Wanted: a love of learning and teaching. After college or university, many adults are eager for new opportunities to learn. They find that there are subject areas they neglected earlier or that they have acquired new interests. There are also those activities and interests for which they now have more time. Student groups are often of special interest to tour guides, because cultural and artistic heritage is not an important priority in most school districts. Museums, on the other hand, are eager to contribute their resources to helping citizens grow in cultural awareness.

The student group that I focus on at present is the high school youth. Here we conduct a set number of tours that have been prepared by the education department of the AGO in conjunction with the docents.

Our docent training is ongoing. It begins with an intense six-week training session, and then the new docents are apprenticed to the AGO regular docents in one of three groups: adult touring, youth/high school, or elementary school children.

Learning takes place by following other docent tours and modeling a tour with a partner until confidence builds, allowing you to go solo. Researching the gallery collection and constant study is ongoing.

One of the best stimulants of the program, I find, is the other docents — a very challenging, fun group of all ages. Docents with a fine arts background, as well as teaching experience, will leap ahead initially. But others who are keen to learn will advance quickly.

New exhibitions at the gallery must be studied in depth and included in existing programs. These existing programs are revamped and reviewed often to keep them fresh and alive. In this way, the docents and their programs continue to be revitalized. Because museums and art galleries are educational institutions, there is a responsibility to provide information about their collections in a credible and interesting way.

The AGO focuses on an interactive approach to learning; the docent involves the viewer in a dialogue or an exercise that entails active looking on the part of the viewer.

Art galleries around the world offer a variety of training programs. In Canada, check with the gallery or museum in your area for information about becoming a docent. If you have acceptable qualifications for the gallery or museum in your area, go for it! If you love art and want an educational challenge, this could be for you. The Art Gallery of Ontario Web site is at www.ago.on.ca.

Fresh Air in Canadian Parks

Imagine spending your volunteer time in the beautiful setting of one of our Canadian parks. Any of our provincial parks would be glad to hear from you. Do a little research in your home province and learn about the volunteer opportunities available. You can participate in such ways as public relations, education and interpretation, photography, scientific studies, research, trail development and maintenance, and administrative support. For further information call the Parks Department in your home province. Visit our Web site at www.after50.ca for Parks Web sites.

Culture Link

Culture Link in Toronto is looking for volunteers to lend a hand to new arrivals to Canada by helping them learn English and reduce their feeling of isolation. Help them to get to know Toronto, their new home. In Metro Toronto, call 416-588-6288.

A similar organization in Regina, the Open Door Society of the Immigrant and Refugee Settlement Agency, is always looking for volunteers. Contact society at: 306-352-3500 or e-mail: rods.host@access-comm.ca. Check for similar organizations in other cities across Canada.

Trust the Weatherman

Did you know that Environment Canada relies on a network of several thousand volunteers across Canada for weather information? It's true! They take daily readings of temperature and precipitation, keep notes on general weather characteristics, and forward monthly reports to Environment Canada. And that's been going on since 1840. The information they gather helps Environment Canada in its continuing study of the weather and climatic fluctuations that affect our everyday lives. Observers include people of all ages from all walks of life: farmers, homemakers, clergy, seniors, and school teachers.

Environment Canada supplies training and equipment and covers the cost of operating expenses. If you are interested in becoming a weather volunteer, contact your local weather office or a regional office of Environment Canada.

Each year, certificates and awards are presented to individuals and families who have reached milestones of long-time service as volunteer climate observers. In the year 2001, 12 Albertans, 17 Manitobans, and 20 Saskatchewanians received awards for their commitment, ranging from 5 to 40 years of service.

Volunteer Opportunities Overseas

Volunteering to help less fortunate people in some distant part of the world is indeed a worthy goal. To provide you with an introduction to the volunteer opportunities available overseas we have provided an overview of four organizations that are active in this field. If you want more information about overseas volunteering, as well as a complete list of volunteering agencies in Canada, check out this Web site: www.citizens4change.org.

CESO — Canadian Executive Service Organization

CESO is a not-for-profit organization offering technical and management expertise to developing and new market economies. CESO volunteers serve as advisers and mentors to enterprises in Canadian First Nation, Metis, and Inuit communities, developing nations around the world, and the new market economies of Central and Eastern Europe and the former Soviet Union. Since its inception in 1967, CESO has completed more than 10,000 assignments worldwide.

Volunteer advisers (VAs) are men and women who are willing and able to apply their years of experience and skills to solving problems in various industries. Most VAs are retired or semi-retired, but many are still professionally active. All must have proven experience to serve as mentors and advisers.

If you are interested in joining CESO or want to obtain more information, please contact the organization in Toronto at: 416-961-2376 ext. 223. Its Web site is at www.ceso-saco.com.

CCI — Canadian Crossroads International

CCI is a unique volunteer-driven organization with more than 700 volunteers worldwide actively involved in all aspects of programming and administrative operations. Participants are matched to a variety of community-based activities run by local non-governmental organizations working to address community needs in the areas of health, education, social development, agriculture, rural development, and the environment. Its Web site is at www.cciorg.ca. Contact Canadian Crossroads International by phone: in Toronto, 416-967-0801; in Montreal, 514-528-5363; in Halifax, 902-422-2933, or in Vancouver, 604-734-4677.

CUSO

CUSO is a Canadian volunteer-sending organization that supports international alliances for social justice and promotes policies for global sustainability. CUSO works with people striving for freedom, gender and racial equality, self-determination, and cultural survival. Approximately 200 CUSO cooperates (international volunteers) are currently on postings with partner organizations in Africa, Asia-Pacific, Latin America, and the Caribbean. Since 1961, CUSO has sent more than 12,000 Canadians overseas. For more information, contact the organization at: CUSO, 500-2255 Carling Avenue, Ottawa, ON, K2B 1A6. Web site: www.cuso.org.

VSO Canada — Voluntary Service Overseas

VSO Canada is a national partner of VSO, the world's largest independent international development agency working through volunteers. Since 1958, more than 29,000 men and women have participated in VSO by sharing their skills alongside people in developing countries, working with them to realize their true potential.

VSO sends professional people, age 21 to 65, to share their skills and experience in education, health, social and community work, business, natural resources, and technical development. Mature volunteers often cite that they appreciate the level of respect they are given as "elders" in other cultures and the value that is placed upon their knowledge and life experience.

For further information, contact Voluntary Service Overseas Canada at 806-151 Slater Street, Ottawa, ON, K1P 5H3; Ph.: 613-234-1364 or 1-888-876-2911. Its Web site is at www.vsocanada.org.

Your Personal Goals

You are now aware of the numerous volunteer opportunities available, from driving for Meals on Wheels to serving on the board of directors of an organization. You have read actual excerpts from organizations seeking volunteers and you are aware of the personal benefits to be derived from volunteering your time and talent. You also know that it is important for you to select a volunteer position that you are comfortable with so that your volunteering experience will be a rewarding one.

The following questionnaire will help you clarify in your own mind exactly what volunteer position you would like to consider. We suggest you complete the questionnaire now while the topic of volunteerism is fresh in your mind.

ACTIVITY # 6: YOUR THOUGHTS ABOUT VOLUNTEERING

1. Thinking of volunteering, is there a social problem or some area of need that you have a special interest in? If so, write a short sentence about it.

2. If you volunteer, what time commitment are you willing to make?

    Daily   _____

    Weekly   _____

    Long Term _____

3. Where would you prefer to work?

    At home   _____

    At another location   _____

4. Name a few of your specific skills or talents.

    *   _____

    *   _____

    *   _____

    *   _____

5. What type of volunteer work would you like to do?

6. What organization would you like to volunteer for?

7. On what date would you be ready to begin as a volunteer?

Make That Phone Call

If you are interested in volunteering, we have made it easy for you to take the next step. There are three ways to make contact with the organization of your choice:

1. If you want to volunteer through a volunteer centre, give the one nearest you a call. You can also contact a volunteer centre if you want further information about volunteering. You can find a list of volunteer centres across Canada on Volunteer Canada's Web site at www.volunteer.ca.

2. If you want to volunteer at a hospital in your area, simply look up the phone number for volunteer services and give them a call.

3. If you want to volunteer for an overseas service contact the appropriate organization by phone or through one of the Web sites we have provided.

QUICK SUMMARY

- Almost one-quarter of the Canadian seniors population volunteer their time and talents in their community. Volunteering has a positive impact on their lives.

- There are eight major categories of organizations that seek volunteers to help them carry out their role in society.

- There are four easy ways to volunteer: contact your local volunteer centre, contact the organization directly, volunteer with VOE over the Internet, or contact Charity Village.

- There are numerous overseas volunteer opportunities.

In this chapter:

- Find out how the computer and the Internet can open doors of opportunity, then decide if it's for you.

- Find out how to make an informed buying decision.

- Find out where to get computer instruction after your purchase.

- Find effective Internet and e-mail training at little or no cost.

"The typewriter has passed the torch to the personal computer and shifted itself to the museums and the history books."

— Madhavi Acharya, *Toronto Star* reporter

This Fascinating Computer Age

Your grandchildren know their way around a computer before they start kindergarten, and 10 year olds toss around terms like megahertz, CD burner, and motherboard with greater ease than many adults. With every passing day more and more seniors lose their fear of the computer and take the plunge into this fascinating world of instant gratification. The Internet is becoming so user friendly that grandparents are now earning university degrees through cyberspace.

The computer is a fascinating piece of equipment that can literally bring the world into your home. With a few clicks of the mouse you can check the weather in Cairo, scan the *Washington Post*, or send an e-mail to a friend in Paris without it costing you a penny extra. If you just want to idle away your time you can play solitaire on your computer screen.

This chapter is directed at members of the 50-plus group who have not been exposed to the wonders of the computer and what it has to offer. If you are seeking something new and different to spice up and enrich your life, give serious thought to bringing a computer into your life. Investing in a computer is not unlike what our parents did when they signed up for electricity, installed a telephone, or purchased a gramophone. In their own way each of these conveniences improved and enhanced the lifestyles of our ancestors.

Make an Informed Decision

We are not suggesting that you rush out and buy a computer. But you owe it to yourself to learn enough about computers that you can make an informed decision about whether to buy or not to buy.

Becoming computer literate can do as much to stimulate your mind as walking or cycling will do to strengthen your body. Check it out, and if your research convinces you that a computer will enrich your life, carefully analyze your needs, learn all you can about what's on the market, and proceed with your purchase. But if after reading this chapter you don't see how the computer could benefit your life, don't go down that road; there are many other ways to challenge your mind. If you have no need for a computer, don't allow yourself to be suckered into buying one, for it will only gather dust and become obsolete and worthless.

You're Being Pressured

Indirectly, there is considerable pressure on everyone — including seniors — to purchase and learn how to use a computer. Soon you will have to tap into the Internet just to get the information you need to function in today's society. Even today, if you want information about what's going on in your own community or an update on weather conditions or medical information, the most efficient way to find that information is to log onto the Internet. The fastest way to send a letter is not via priority post, it's over the Internet via e-mail. The computer and the Internet are here to stay. The least you can do is evaluate the pros and cons of computer ownership. Don't dismiss that possibility without finding out what it has to offer. You are never too old. I was 62 when I bought my first Macintosh with that tiny screen. That may have been the most significant purchase I ever made, because since then it has had a huge positive impact on my life.

Statistics: Where Do You Fit In?

The following excerpts are taken from Statistics Canada's General Social Survey, 2000. The GSS is an annual telephone sample survey. This survey focused on the use and impact of computer and Internet technology on Canadians. The sample had 25,090 respondents. This is the first time Statistics Canada collected detailed information on individual use of technology.

What follows is only a fraction of the information contained in Heather Dryburgh's analysis of Statistics Canada's survey entitled, "Changing Our Ways: Why and How Canadians Use the Internet." Unfortunately the report concentrates on individuals who use the Internet with barely any mention of those who own a computer but are not on the Internet.

Half of Us Are On the Net

An estimated 13 million — 53 percent of Canadians over 15 years of age — used the Internet in the 12 months prior to the survey. Approximately 50 percent of women use the Internet, compared to 56 percent of men. Here is a breakdown of Internet usage by age categories. Note that Internet usage declines steadily for each subsequent age group.

- 90 percent of teens aged 15 to 19 use the Internet.
- 70 percent of individuals aged 25 to 29 use the Internet.
- 61 percent of individuals aged 35 to 39 use the Internet.
- 13 percent of seniors aged 65 to 69 use the Internet.

How We Use the Internet

- 61 percent use the Internet from 1 to 7 hours per week.
- 14 percent use the Internet at home for more than 14 hours per week.
- 55 percent use the Internet to access on-line news sites.
- 50 percent use the Internet to search for health and medical information.
- 56 percent search the Internet for entertainment and sports information.
- About 84 percent of Internet users are connected to e-mail and many (39 percent) use it as a daily communication tool.

The Computer, A Catalyst for Change

In the 50-plus age group you'll find that the computer and the Internet offer countless opportunities for a turnaround in your lifestyle. Suddenly you can experience the exhilaration of immediate feedback from your own work, a renewed interest in daily life, and a sense of personal accomplishment you don't want to miss. If you are searching for an active mind, here are some of the ways the computer will make that possible.

- **To correspond with family and friends.** You can send and receive personal e-mail letters to family and friends at no additional cost. And best of all there is no waiting time for delivery; your e-mail arrives at the other end in an instant. Sure there is a cost for the Internet service, but it gives you access 24 hours a day, 7 days a week to anywhere in the world for free. You can even send family pictures and documents attached to your e-mail.
- **To write your memoirs.** If you get the urge to put your personal life onto paper there's no better way to do it than via the computer. When you write by hand, you either get it right the first time or you start all over again. Not so with the computer; you can make all the changes and corrections you want.

Write a little bit every day and soon you will be amazed at what you have accomplished.

- **To record family history information.** Genealogy software programs are available for this purpose and there are numerous sites on the Internet that offer assistance in getting started and finding information. See Chapter 8: Tracing Your Ancestors for more information.

- **To research a hobby.** On the Internet, you can find information on any topic you can think of. If your hobby is stamp collecting, sports, or learning about the solar system, you will find dozens of Web sites devoted to your special interest. Once on the Internet, the world is literally at your fingertips. If you have an interest in a particular subject, explore the vast repository of data that's available to all of us on the Internet. Why not open that window and take a look inside?

- **To further your education.** Whether you want to take a full university degree course or enroll in one or more sessions of continuing education, that opportunity is available over the Internet. The number of universities and other institutions offering on-line education is on the increase. The opportunities for on-line learning are endless and the number of grandparents enrolling is rising. You will find more on that subject in Chapter 9: The Learning Journey.

- **To get the news.** Are you one of those people who just can't get enough news? You can get local and world news 24 hours a day. If you're on the Internet you no longer have to buy a dozen papers every day to satisfy your craving. You can read every major newspaper in the world over the Internet. If you're a doubting Thomas, take a look at the CEO Express Web site: www.ceoexpress.com.

- **To get weather information.** For information about Canada or anywhere in the world, take a look at these two sites. Weather is important if you're planning a trip, and now it's available with a few clicks of the mouse. World Weather is at www.worldweather.com. The Canadian Weather Office Web site is at www.weatheroffice.com.

- **To research your vacation destination.** Click here for the best of Canada on-line, everything from Canadian hotels to Canadian highways: www.discovercanada.com. For world coverage try: www.cities.com. It's easy to navigate and provides a comprehensive description of more than 4,300 cities in 150 countries.
- **To carry out volunteer work for various organizations.** Yes, some organizations depend upon their volunteers to do work that involves using the computer and the Internet.
- **To play computer games.** There are computer games on the market for every age group and every level of difficulty.
- **To do your personal banking.** Not only can you do your personal banking on-line, you can now pay many of your bills on-line as well.
- **To record your investments.** Again, several companies specialize in producing computer software expressly designed for recording your investments. You can check out the various programs on the market at your local computer store.
- **To get medical information.** There are hundreds of Web sites with medical information on the Internet. While some sources are said to be unreliable, you can always feel comfortable with our own Health Canada site, which can be found at www.hc-sc.gc.ca. You can search Health Canada's site for information about a specific disease, medication, treatment, or illness.

A second excellent site is provided by the National Library of Medicine in the U.S. at www.medlineplus.gov. It has an first-rate medical dictionary, includes information about diseases and drugs, as well as informative articles on exercise and fitness.

According to a new survey, next to face-to-face contact with a health professional, the Internet is the most common means for Canadians to get health information, ranking ahead of radio, television, and newspapers.

Ah! The Downside

The computer brings with it at least three concerns you should be aware of:

1. A computer along with the required monitor, printer, and software does cost money, so be prepared for the expenditure. The price you pay will depend upon your individual needs. At the time of writing you can purchase a high-quality system, including monitor and printer, for less than $2,000.

2. Getting hooked on the computer has the potential to confine you to a sedentary lifestyle that is totally contrary to what we have advocated in Part One of this book. Therefore you have an obligation to yourself to maintain a balance in your life. Pull yourself away from the computer periodically to get your daily exercise. It can be done, all it takes is willpower.

3. Operating a computer calls for more than flipping a switch. You have to learn how to use it. But don't be scared off; it's not that difficult. We'll delve into the degree of difficulty and how to get instruction later on. In any case, learning new things is what keeps your brain alive.

Before You Buy

Can't Type? Don't Worry.

Legend has it that some of the speediest newspaper reporters used only two or maybe four fingers to do their typing, and that may be the route you want to follow. If it's your ambition to type like a pro, using all ten fingers, there are several typing software programs on the market, such as Typing Tutor, that promise better and faster typing. Whatever method you use, the more you type the better you'll become. If you are a novice at the keyboard, don't worry about your typing errors; word processing programs generally come with great spell-checking systems.

A Bit of Homework

If you've got the urge to purchase your first computer there are two things you should do beforehand:

- Familiarize yourself with computer terminology, and
- Get some hands-on experience with a computer.

But don't hold back because you don't know how it works. In recent years the computer has truly become user friendly, and you can learn the basics in a few hours of instruction. Remember, you don't need to know how a computer works to operate one. You have been using the telephone and television for years, and if you are like the vast majority of the population you haven't the faintest idea how they work. You probably drive a car, but you're not a mechanic. The point is that you need to know only how to operate a computer, not how it works.

There are several ways to acquire your know-how. The best way for you will depend on:

- how much money you want to spend,
- how you like to learn, and
- how much time you have.

Try Your Local Library

Most libraries now have personal computers (PCs) available for use by their members. These computers, usually equipped with Microsoft Word and other programs, are available to patrons at no charge. This is a great way for potential computer buyers to get hands-on practice without any investment.

Many libraries also have computers dedicated to Internet access. Here is your opportunity to get acquainted with the Internet. Although library staff do not have time to provide detailed instruction, they will get you started and then you can take it from there. There is no cost, but there may be a time limit.

Have Someone on Your Side

Before buying a computer seek out a "computer literate" friend or family member who can answer your questions and explain basic computer terminology. Ask this person to explain the purpose of the major components and what makes one computer better than another. One of the first things your computer literate friend will probably ask is: "What are you going to use your computer for?" Once that question is answered it will be much easier for both of you to make the right buying decision.

A computer is made up of numerous components, each manufactured by a different company with significant differences in quality and efficiency. What initially appears to be a good deal may only reflect the fact that the lower-priced computer contains inexpensive components. Apply the same thought process to your purchase of a printer and monitor. Find out what makes one product better than another.

If you are dealing with a smaller company, find out how long they have been in business and inquire about warranty, service, and telephone support. A good way to learn about a company is to visit its corporate Web site; you would be surprised what information you can find out. A good in-depth Web site is often a good indicator that they know their stuff.

So Many Choices

There are so many arrangements of computer specifications and prices that it appears almost impossible to make that so-called wise buying decision. There are starter kits as low as $499 and high-performance packages at $2,999. So take the time to learn the basics about computers, find an "advisor" friend, or seek out an informed salesperson at a reliable computer store who is willing to help.

Ask your consultant friend to accompany you on a visit to two or three computer stores. Talk with computer salespeople and get prices on some of their products. With this approach you will make a more informed decision and feel more comfortable with your purchase than if you make the purchase blindly on your own. Computer salespeople are notorious for using technical jargon, so it's in your best interests to have someone on your side to translate computer lingo into plain English.

Good Value

When you buy a computer, printer, or monitor today you are getting much more for your money than you would have last year or five years ago. While you may pay $2,000 to get established with everything you need to get up and running, your computer will be more user friendly and faster than anyone dreamed possible several years ago.

You should also be aware that the computer industry is in a constant state of flux with new products, faster speeds, and more memory. As a result, your new computer becomes obsolete the moment you take it out of the box. There is always something new and better, but as long as the product you purchased meets your needs, you have no cause for concern. The day may come eventually, of course, when your computer is no longer compatible with new software programs, which are also upgraded every few months.

Computer First, Internet Later

If you are new to computers, don't purchase your computer and arrange for Internet hook-up at the same time. Leave an adjustment period of at least one month between the purchase of your first computer and your Internet hook-up. If you do otherwise, the whole process will be extremely overwhelming and it will take the enjoyment out of both purchases. First get your computer, monitor, and printer set up and installed. Learn how to use the computer, and once you feel comfortable with that first step, proceed with the Internet hook-up.

A Computer for You

The first question is whether to buy a PC (Personal Computer) or a Macintosh. The PC is the logical choice for first-time buyers because it's the favourite for about 90 percent of the personal computer market. PCs use an operating system called Microsoft Windows, which is compatible with most software and is what most people use. If at some time in the future you begin doing specialized work such as desktop publishing or graphics you may decide to get a Macintosh, as it is strong in these areas.

Now that you know you are looking for a PC, don't ignore the possibility of purchasing a used computer. There are a lot of good buys out there, and it is an affordable alternative.

Get the Package

Most retailers offer a packaged system that includes the computer and a monitor, various software, and sometimes a printer. Some offer a range of packages whereby for a little more money you can get larger capacity, more features, and better components. Buying a package like this usually ends up being less costly than buying each item separately. What you decide to purchase (with the help of your advisor or salesperson) will depend upon the size of your wallet and what you intend to use your computer for. Much like buying a car, you can often select various options for the package. But keep in mind, these options will directly effect the end price.

As of December 2002, you can purchase a powerful Intel Pentium 4, 2.53 GHz computer with 512 MBs of RAM, an 80 GB hard drive, a CD rewriter, and many other extras in a package that includes a monitor, printer, and software for less than $2,000. This is a great value for your money. With the fast-paced changes in the computer world, you will probably get even more for your dollar by the time you read this.

When you look at the numbers presented in this section, be aware that there are 1,000 kilobytes (KB) in a megabyte (MB), and 1,000 megabytes in a gigabyte (GB).

The Major Components

The CPU

The CPU (Central Processing Unit) is basically the brain of the computer system. It processes instructions and carries out the commands you give your computer. When I purchased my Intel Pentium 3 computer less than two years ago it came with a speed of 800 MHz (megahertz). At the time of writing the Intel Pentium 4 runs at much faster speeds, in the range of 2.50 GHz plus, and the price is lower. Emphasis is placed on the numbers because the higher the gigahertz rating, the quicker the computer will process your information. Do we need all this speed? Probably not, unless you are heavily into games, videos, artwork, or desktop publishing.

Early on in your purchasing search you will be forced to decide between four processors: Intel's Pentium or its budget line Celeron, or AMD's Athlon or its budget line Duron. Each of these processors has its own features and benefits. Which one you choose will depend upon your particular needs, including how much you want to spend. To insure satisfaction, get a computer with a fairly fast processor, such as the 2.53 GHz in this package.

One computer authority had this to say about processors: "Higher speed budget chips can now handle demanding software. The AMD Athlon and the Duron have both beaten the equivalent Intel chips in some speed trials."

Currently the CPUs available on the market run in what is called a 32-bit architecture. Just over the horizon looms the new 64-bit processor. It will certainly be a revolution in the computing industry. It may already be available by the time you read this chapter.

RAM

RAM (Random Access Memory) is usually measured in megabytes (MB) and has a direct influence on the speed of your system. Less than two years ago the standard for RAM was 128 MB; today it's four times that at 512 MB. RAM is the temporary data storage area in your computer. It holds all the programs and data you have open at one time. RAM is only active when your computer is in use. The more RAM you have, the more files and programs you can have open at any one time. Once you turn your computer off, everything stored in RAM disappears. Increasing the memory in your computer is an inexpensive way to boost your computer's power, so purchase the most you can afford.

Hard Drive

The hard disk drive is your computer's permanent electronic filling cabinet. It stores your operating system, your programs, and all your files. A while back, the standard hard drive had 30 gigabytes (GB) of space; today it's much larger. Since most new software programs require large amounts of storage, hard drive space can fill up rather quickly. Text does not take up much space, but photographs and some computer programs do. For instance, one page of text takes up only about 20 KB (kilobytes). This whole book uses only about 5 MB of space. If you had a 40 GB hard drive, it would hold 8,000 books like this one.

CD-ROM and/or DVD Drive

Most new computers sold these days come with a CD-ROM drive. It is simply a drive that reads data from a disk or CD (compact disk). A CD-ROM drive can also play music CDs as long as it is connected to a sound card and a set of speakers.

The current industry trend is leaning heavily towards the DVD drive. It can do everything a CD-ROM drive can do plus it can play DVD movies right on your computer. As many new programs get larger in size, companies will soon be shifting towards the DVD as the preferred method of distribution. In terms of capacity, a DVD holds six times the data of a CD and there are new processes in the works that are trying to push that limit. Thus, you will see the DVD drive often as you seek out your purchase.

CD-Rewriter

Also known as a CD burner, the CD-Rewriter allows you to transfer text, photographs, and other data from your computer onto a blank writeable CD. It is an especially useful feature for backing up your work. It is also a great way to share your files and photographs with family, friends, and colleagues.

Sound Card

It's the sound card that allows your computer to reproduce sounds, voices, and music. When you hear that sound telling you that you have received new e-mail it's the sound card at work.

Video Card

The video card (often referred to as a graphics card or display adapter) is partly responsible for what you see on your screen. It translates what the processor produces into a form that the monitor can display. The most important specification with a video card is its RAM rating. At the time of this writing the industry standard for video card size is 64 MB.

Modem

The most important function of the modem is to put your computer "on-line," that is, to connect it to the Internet. If you want to be connected you must have a modem. There are a variety of modems and corresponding services to accommodate this need.

The basic telephone line connection uses a standard modem, which offers speeds up to 56 Kbps (kilobits per second). Your computer must have this type of modem in order to get on-line through telephone lines. The two other choices in the mainstream are DSL and cable modems, which are rented to you by your service provider.

The DSL service uses your standard phone line, but provides much faster service and uses a special "always on" modem. The cable modem allows your computer to connect to the Internet via your cable TV system. Both of these high-speed modems offer speeds well in excess of the standard 56 K modem. One drawback to these high-speed services is that they are not yet available everywhere, but that too is rapidly changing.

Keyboard and Mouse

You must have a way to tell the computer what you want it to do. This is where the mouse and the keyboard come into play. When computers first appeared on the scene, executives rebelled at getting their fingers too close to the keyboard. How demeaning! That's what secretaries did at their typewriters. But that all changed when some bright fellow introduced the term "keying in" to describe what has always been called "typing." Now, senior executives key in much of their own correspondence, but of course they never type.

The mouse is a graphical device that allows you to point to areas of the computer screen to initiate a task, whether it is to launch a program or to click a button to send an e-mail. If you don't like the speed of your mouse, find out how to adjust the mouse settings so that the touch feels comfortable as you use it.

Software

The term "software" refers to the programs that allow you to do such things as write letters, enter data, and perform calculations on your computer. There are hundreds of software programs available for a large variety of needs. Your choice of software will be determined by what kind of work you do on your computer. The two programs you will most likely need are Microsoft Word, for writing letters, reports etc., and Microsoft Excel, a spreadsheet program in which you can enter numbers into a grid of rows and columns and perform calculations.

If you get involved with genealogy you will want to investigate and purchase a genealogy software program. If you are interested in photography you may want to consider photo editing software. Certainly one of the first programs you should purchase is an anti-virus protection program.

Monitor

It is through the monitor that the computer communicates with you and provides that instant gratification that we all love so much. Most monitors today have a standard 17-inch screen. But there is a gradual trend to larger 19-inch monitors, which call for more desk space and more money. Flat screens are also available for a few more dollars. A flat screen is said to reduce glare and distortion and therefore be easier on the eyes. When buying a monitor you should also be interested in picture quality. One of the important criteria is the "dot pitch." The lower the dot pitch the crisper the image.

Colour Printer

A printer attached to your system is essential if you want to have a hard (paper) copy of the work you produce. A colour printer allows you to print out text or photographs in brilliant colour. Check out the prices and you'll find that printers are quite inexpensive these days. One of the drawbacks of regular printers is the ongoing cost of ink cartridges. The alternative is to purchase a laser printer, but the initial cost is considerably higher.

Instruction after the Purchase

Here are six ways to learn how to use the computer and the Internet after you have made the purchase and have a computer in your home.

1. Self-Instruction

The most inexpensive method is to combine periodic instruction from a friend or family member with plenty of practice and self-instruction. Going this route requires self-discipline because the only learning deadlines you will have are those you impose upon yourself. This method also requires that you do considerable reading and find your own answers to your computer questions. Two of your best sources for this information are computer reference books and the extensive "Help" files that come with your software.

If you search the bookstores and computer stores you will find excellent "teach yourself" books. Some even come with instruction and lesson plans on a CD.

2. Creative Retirement Computer Club

The Creative Retirement Computer Club (CRCC) in Winnipeg has offered computer courses to older adults for years. Its on-line course, "Guide to Computing," includes how to buy a PC, understanding and using a computer, a glossary of terms, and a guide to computer components.

Go to the club's Web site at www.seniorscan.ca, click on "Computer Club" or "Guide to Computing" and you will find all the information you need for free. Regardless of where you live, there is probably a seniors' computer training group in progress right now.

3. Techno Tips

Techno Tips is just one of the offerings from Ryerson's on-line Senior Centre. In addition to constantly updated hints and tricks it offers a comprehensive on-line computer training program. Help yourself by visiting the Techno Tips Web site at www.seniorcentre.ca/docs/computer.html

4. SeniorNet

SeniorNet in the U.S. caters to the 50-plus group by providing education and training in various parts of the States. You will find interesting discussions about the computer and the Internet at its Web site: www.seniornet.org/php.

5. Computer Classroom Instruction

Computer training is available from a wide variety of sources in every community. Listed below are suggestions of places to check. As you conduct your comparison shopping, be aware that many computer training companies offer a discount for seniors. Also keep in mind that most courses on a subject such as Microsoft Word are delivered at three levels: introductory, intermediate, and advanced. Therefore, to get the full training on a specific topic you may require three courses. Some training sources are:

- your local district school board,
- community colleges,
- community centres, and
- senior centres.

6. On-line Training

There is an increasing trend towards delivering educational programs over the Internet. On-line training is not for everyone, but it does have a number of advantages. It is less costly than classroom training and you can study at your own pace whenever you wish. If you select on-line training, set your own personal achievement goals and see them through. If you are interested in on-line computer training explore what these Web sites have to offer:

- The Brookeline Internet & Computer Services Inc., Victoria, B.C. This company offers a wide range of computer and related on-line training courses. See its Web site at www.trainingontheweb.net.
- The University of Waterloo in Waterloo, Ontario offers a complete line of computer training over the Internet in what it calls distance education. Don't miss its site at http://dce.uwaterloo.ca.
- The University of Calgary in Calgary, Alberta offers a computer training program for seniors on location at the university. It also offers a variety of regular computer training on-line. Its Web site is at www.ucalgary.ca/cted/compuofc.

The Internet

One Internet service provider (ISP) described the Internet this way: "The Internet is a global network of networks that connects thousands of computer systems, and millions of users together in one globally oriented information resource." The most amazing aspect of the Internet is that nobody owns it and most of its services are free.

Find Your ISP

Your first step in getting hooked up to the Internet is to select an Internet service provider (ISP). There are thousands of ISPs across the country. They sell access to the Internet by providing the technological link that allows your computer to connect to the millions of Web sites around the world. Your ISP connects your computer to the World Wide Web and provides the technology for you to send and receive e-mail.

Depending on your choice of service, your ISP hook-up to the Internet will be in any one of the following ways:

- a dial-up connection over regular telephone lines,
- a cable modem service from a cable TV company, or
- a DSL (digital subscriber line) service from a phone company.

For years, the traditional method of hooking up to the Internet was via regular telephone lines. With this system, if you have a single telephone line connection, your phone is not available for normal use when you are on-line. That's quite a disadvantage. But now there are alternatives.

High-Speed Service

If you want high-speed service you have three choices: a cable connection with your local cable company, a DSL hook-up from your phone company, or a wireless high-speed service. They will all give you a permanent Internet connection, which means that your computer is always on-line. These high-speed connections also free up your phone line.

This faster Internet service is about twice as costly as a regular telephone line connection. In the fall of 2002, high-speed service was priced at about $50 a month. Since cable and DSL connections are permanent you no longer have to dial up your ISP to get on-line, and the extra speed provides instant connection when moving from one Web site to another. You have to decide whether the additional speed is worth the added cost to you.

What to Look for in an ISP

If you are not in a hurry, there are hundreds of smaller local ISPs that provide traditional telephone dial-up service. It's important to find a reliable ISP that will provide the service you are entitled to. Without a doubt, the best way to find the right ISP is to seek out recommendations from your friends and neighbours. Here are some of the things to look for, and to look out for, when deciding on your ISP:

- As with any purchase decision, do adequate comparison shopping.
- Get recommendations from friends and relatives.
- Make sure it is a local phone call to your ISP. You don't want

to be hit with long-distance phone costs every time you dial up for a connection.

- Ask for the ISP's range of rates for Internet access, then decide upon the best choice for your needs. Packages range from 15 hours per month for as little as $6.95, to unlimited monthly access for as little as $19.95.
- Make sure your ISP provides all the software necessary to connect your computer to the Internet.
- Make sure there is no set-up charge.
- Make sure the ISP provides good technical support — most do.
- Verify that you can get their tech support on the phone without a lengthy delay. Call them. How long was your wait time?
- Obtain assurance from other users that you can connect to the Internet at will without encountering frequent busy signals.
- Find out if you can enroll for a trial period before making a long-term commitment.

Searching the World Wide Web

Once connected to your ISP, you will use a software program called a browser to search through the myriad of documents called "Web pages" stored on computers around the world. The two most popular browsers are Netscape Navigator and Microsoft Internet Explorer. Essentially, there are two ways to find information on the Internet:

1. If you know the Web page address, or URL as it is called, of the site you want to visit, you can easily type in the address, and the browser will display the Web site on your screen. A URL will look something like this: http://www.microsoft.com/download. Once a site is open you can view all sorts of data contained on that Web site and possibly click your way to other linked sites. The speed at which the pages open and the speed at which you can browse from one Web site to another distinguishes high-speed access from the conventional dial-up connection.

2. Your other option is to search for a URL using a search engine. A search engine can help you find the URL of a specific company or organization, or it can give you a list of URLs on any given topic that interests you. Let's say you wanted to search for information about castles in Scotland. You would enter the words "Castles Scotland" in the search box of your favourite search engine, click on "Go," and bingo, you will be presented with hundreds of "finds" to select from. Search engines are essential to any kind of research. Some well-known search engines are: Yahoo, Google, Infoseek, Excite, Lycos, and AltaVista. Each search engine has its own characteristics and its own group of followers. Here is a brief sampling you can try out.

    *   Yahoo is at http://www.yahoo.com (also Yahoo Canada at: http://ca.yahoo.com).
    *   Google is at: http://www.google.com (also Google Canada at: http://www.google.ca).
    *   AltaVista's Web site is http://www.altavista.com.
    *   Search.com searches out other search engines and always finds numerous good hits. You'll find it at: http://www.search.com.
    *   Metacrawler also calls upon several other search engines to do the search work. Visit: http://www.metacrawler.com.

Here Are a Few Interesting Web Sites to Get You Started

*   A Canadian phone directory site: http://canada411.sympatico.ca
*   CBC news site: http://cbc.ca/news
*   Canoe, a Canadian news site: http://www.canoe.ca
*   The Canadian government welcomes you to Seniors Canada On-line: http://www.seniors.gc.ca
*   The Canadian Seniors Policies and Programs Database by province: http://www.sppd.gc.ca

- Discover Canada, a site devoted to great travel destinations within Canada: http://www.discovercanada.com
- The SeniorsCan Internet Program (SCIP) is an exceptional guide for retirees and older adults in all of Canada. Don't miss it! Visit: http://www.seniorscan.ca.
- Our own Web site is at http://www.after50.ca. We invite you to visit it, for it contains a host of Web site links and other information you will be interested in.

Send and Receive E-mail

Once you are hooked up to an Internet service provider you are ready to begin sending and receiving electronic mail, commonly called e-mail. Your e-mail program may already be installed in your computer. If not, you can download one for free. The most common e-mail programs are Outlook Express, Eudora, and Netscape.

E-mail is a short and snappy way to communicate, and for some reason it invites informality. For instance, most people use the salutation "Hi Joan" rather than "Dear Joan." It seems perfectly correct and proper when in the e-mail format. Despite that informality, electronic communication does have its own rules of etiquette. For example:

- Don't send a message in all capital letters. Not only is it hard to read, it's interpreted as shouting.
- Always enter the subject of your communication in the subject line of your e-mail.

Working with your provider you will decide upon a user name, your ID. Oftentimes your user name will in some way be a reflection of your own name. If your first name is Joanne and your Internet service provider is Bell Canada's Sympatico, your e-mail address might be joanne@sympatico.ca. The symbol @ is pronounced "at" and the word "sympatico" is the domain name of the ISP. As a rule, there are no spaces between parts of an e-mail address, although there may be hyphens or underscores, and letters are usually lowercase. Our e-mail address is: jim.olga@after50.ca. The "after50" part is based on our Web site address, www.after50.ca.

When someone sends you an e-mail it goes directly to your Internet service provider where it is retained until you go on-line to check your mail. At that time, a list of your new messages appear like magic on your screen. As you click on each message it opens instantaneously, ready to read and then be saved, deleted, or replied to, as you wish.

Your e-mail program contains a variety of neat features that contribute to its usefulness and makes it convenient and easy to use. Some of them are:

Instant Reply: A click on the "Reply" button will set up a new e-mail to respond to one you have received. The new e-mail will appear addressed to the sender of the original e-mail, it will have the original subject line, and the original message will be shown in the body of the new e-mail. If your reply does not relate to the original message, save the reader time by deleting his or her original message from your reply.

Address Book: Your e-mail program will include an address book that can conveniently store the addresses of people with whom you correspond frequently. It's easy to add or delete names from your address book.

Send a Message: To send a message simply click on the name of the person you are sending the message to and your program automatically fills in the e-mail address for that person. You enter the subject, write your message, and click "Send." It's that simple.

Multiple Addresses: If you want to send the same message to many people, simply click the names of all the intended recipients and they will all receive the message. You always know if a message has been sent because sent messages are automatically saved in the "Sent Items" folder.

Folders: It is always a good idea to keep your documents and e-mails well organized. To help you do that, go to File>Folder to create a new folder. Better yet, create several folders so that you can keep related messages together. For example you may have messages related to Activities, Family, and Medical. Give your folders a brief descriptive name and begin moving messages into their appropriate folders. Later, you can delete any files and folders that you no longer need. It is also very easy to change the name of a folder. Check your Help file or refer to one of your reference books to learn how to do it.

Attach a File: Once you get comfortable sending e-mails you may have reason to attach a file to your e-mail. The file could be anything from a report to a picture presently saved in another part of your computer. If you are using Outlook Express, for instance, all you have to do is click the paper clip symbol on the toolbar to bring up the attachment dialogue box. Then, browse to find the file you want to attach to your message, click on the file's name, and send your message. One of the major advantages of using the "attach" option is that documents sent as an attachment retain their formatting. Conversely, when you copy and paste a document into the body of an e-mail message, it does not retain its formatting.

Spell Check: Yes, you can now spell check your e-mail. You can even make it happen automatically for all e-mails you send. Go to Tools>Options>Spelling and place a check mark opposite "Always check spelling before sending," then sit back and rest easy that your message will be letter perfect.

Internet Instruction for the Beginner

At no cost, the following excellent Web sites will provide you with detailed instruction on how to navigate the Internet, use e-mail, and other related topics.

- Beginners Central at: http://northernwebs.com/bc
- The Help Web: http://www.imaginarylandscape.com/helpweb

ACTIVITY # 7: A COMPUTER IN MY LIFE?

1. Circle the number that represents how strongly you want to own a computer and get on the Internet.

   No   Strong
   Desire   Desire
     1   2   3   4   5   6   7   8   9   10

2. If you had a computer in your home with Internet access, state some of the ways you would put it to good use.

3. List some of the steps you can take right now to prepare yourself for your computer purchase.

4. Make a note of other thoughts you have regarding a computer purchase.

QUICK SUMMARY

- Keep an open mind about computers and the Internet. Learn enough about them that you can make an informed buying decision.

- If you are looking for something new and stimulating in your life, owning a computer and getting on the Internet may open a new world of opportunity for you.

- Learning how to use a computer is easier than you think, and there are dozens of ways to receive instruction.

In this chapter:

- Learn where and how to gather family information and how to organize and record it.

- Learn how to put logical time parameters around your research goals.

- Find out where to look for genealogy computer software programs and how to decide which one to buy.

- Learn how to organize your data, put it into book format, and share it with your kin.

Genealogy brings families together.

Family History

Call it genealogy, family history, or a family tree — close to half of North American adults want to make a connection with their past. It caught on in the late seventies after Alex Haley's novel *Roots* appeared on television. Many thousands pursue the search for their ancestors with a passion unlike anything else they have ever tackled. For many, it's a constant search for one more fact, one more name, or one more document. It must be the detective in us that spurs us on to pursue the search and unravel the mysteries so inherent in family history research.

My Seven-Year Stint

I got the bug shortly after I qualified as a senior citizen. I worked on both my father's side and my mother's side simultaneously as I rushed to complete the research, organize the information, write the books, and get them out to my relatives before my Exit time. First I self-published a 400-page genealogy of my father's ancestors in *Out of Bornish*. (Bornish is in the Outer Hebrides of Scotland.) Later I completed *North & South of the 49th*, the family history of my mother's Griffith ancestors.

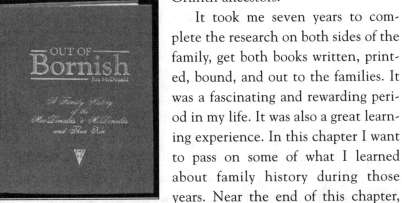

It took me seven years to complete the research on both sides of the family, get both books written, printed, bound, and out to the families. It was a fascinating and rewarding period in my life. It was also a great learning experience. In this chapter I want to pass on some of what I learned about family history during those years. Near the end of this chapter, under the heading "Get It Between the Covers," I discuss the process of how to get a family history into book format. I'm sure you will find it helpful when the time comes for you to take on a similar task.

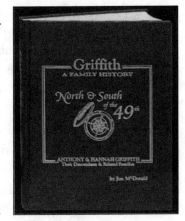

Feedback Is Rewarding

After you have spent years preparing a family history, the members of your extended family appreciate the opportunity to acquire all that research nicely organized into a book ready for reading. When they receive the book containing the history and pictures of their family and their ancestors they are overjoyed, and many take the time to say thank you. Thank-you notes are rewarding, and I have had the good fortune to receive my share. I want you to have a preview of what your feedback may look like, so I have included excerpts from several of the notes I received in response to the Griffith book in the "Feedback" sidebars.

Exciting Moments

Whenever you research the history of a family you are bound to have a few moments of excitement that spur you on just when you have reached a low point in your enthusiasm. Here are three examples from my experience:

- For years I had been searching for a document called a "Declaration of Intent," which may or may not have been completed by my great-grandfather after he arrived in the U.S. If it existed, it would provide evidence of when he arrived as well as other valuable data. After months of waiting, the declaration document finally arrived in the mail and it contained even more information than I expected. That was an exciting moment in the life of this researcher.

- I knew that I had numerous relatives in the U.S. but despite searching through all the normal channels I was unable to locate even one. There were many with the surname Griffith, but they did not match my ancestry. In desperation I took Griffith addresses off the Internet and mailed out a form letter to 100 people in 2 states with that surname. I heard nothing for two months, then I received an e-mail from the U.S. that started out, "I'm your cousin Bill…" That e-mail opened the floodgates to dozens of kin south of the 49th and a family reunion. Another great day.

- I had been searching for a picture of my grandfather Barney for some time. Everyone said, "There's no picture of Grandpa." Then one afternoon I received a call from a cousin in Watrous, Saskatchewan. She said, "We have had a large portrait of Grandpa Barney hanging in the living room for years. Would you like me to send you a copy?" Now that was great news.

Now you have an idea of why people search out their ancestors. Most of the time you get small rewards that keep you going from day to day, but interspersed here and there you get some big ones, too. Family history research is a rewarding endeavor that you may like to pursue. It's one more area of interest that you may want to take up in your quest for a way to maintain an active mind.

This chapter will tell you how to get started, where to look for information, how to get the information, how to organize your information, and how to put it together in the form of a book. Genealogy is a huge subject, so this chapter will only scratch the surface, perk your curiosity, and point you in the right direction. It may be the very thing to fill that void in your life.

Who Are You Researching?

So you are about to embark on a search for your ancestors. Congratulations, but hold on for a moment while you clarify in your own mind exactly who you want to search for. You have two parents, four grandparents, eight great-grandparents, and the numbers keep multiplying the further back you go. If you are married, your spouse has exactly the same kind of lineage. It can be a jungle of people back there in years gone by, so one of the first things you must do is develop a plan and decide which family line you want to search. Here are some early questions you have to answer.

1. Do you want to research your side of the family or your spouse's side?

2. Assume you are going to confine your search to your side of the family only. The next question is, are you going to research your father's side or your mother's side of the family?

Your decision does not have to be as cut and dried as "my father's side only" or "my mother's side only." You can research both your mother's and father's lineage at the same time, but your task will be much more demanding. If you research both your mother's and father's ancestry at the same time, it is absolutely necessary that you keep separate files for each.

 Feedback

Dear Jim,
Many thanks for an excellent epic work! The Griffith book is more massive than I expected ... means there are/were so many of us.
Grace Jerome

The Ancestors Chart

It will be much easier for you to come to a decision about what part of your family you want to research if you begin by creating an ancestors chart. Start by getting a bird's-eye view of what you already know about your ancestors, without the clutter of cousins, uncles, nieces, and nephews. To do that, complete what you presently know about your ancestors on an ancestors or pedigree chart.

An ancestors chart is a graphic documentation that begins with one person and moves backward in time, showing the parents of each person in the tree. The layout of an ancestors chart is shown on the following page. This chart creates a direct line from you to your father and mother and then to your grandparents, great-grandparents and so forth.

ACTIVITY # 8:

1. On a large sheet of paper copy the format of the chart provided to create your own ancestors chart.

2. Enter the names of your parents, the names of their parents, grandparents, and so forth as far back as you can go using information presently available to you.

3. Jot down known dates of birth, marriage, and death wherever you can.

4. Now sit back and take a look at what you already know about your ancestors.

Are you fairly well informed about your ancestors or do you see numerous holes in your information? What you see on your roughed-out ancestors chart will give you a good idea of the extent of the task that lies ahead.

Ancestors Chart Layout

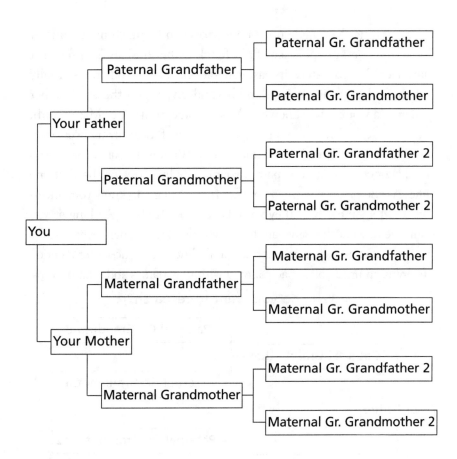

Narrowing the Search

The following chart is a depiction of your father's ancestry only, taken from the larger chart above. If you are going to confine your research to your father's line you have yet another decision to make. Do you want to restrict your search to your male line of ancestors (father, grandfather, great-grandfather) and their wives, brothers, and sisters? Or, do you also want to search your paternal grandmother's line?

Searching the female line of ancestors can be much more difficult due to the common practice of a wife taking her husband's surname at marriage. Unfortunately, in past generations, many women essentially lost their identity at marriage and beyond. Even after the death of her husband, a woman was known as Mrs. George Smith, not Mary Smith.

Many researchers attempt to trace as many of their direct ancestors as possible, from both male and female lines. Whatever your decision, you should concentrate on one part of your family line (tree or chart) at one time. As you progress with your research you will get to know your ancestors and remember how they are related to each other. As long as you continue to work the same family line you will know where everyone fits in, but once you switch to another family line you'll encounter a period of confusion until you get acquainted with new names and relationships.

Who do you want to research?

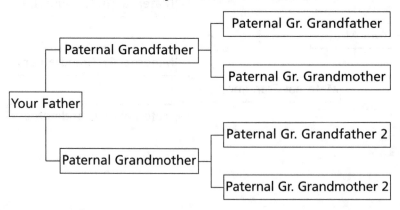

Let us assume that your main interest is in learning about the first ancestor on your father's side to arrive in North America. I say North America because you may not know whether he first landed in Canada or the United States. To avoid confusion, let's put that in the form of a goal statement:

Is this your research goal?
Immediately begin a search for the first ancestor of my father's family line to immigrate to North America.

The example goal statement may be typical of what most people set out to accomplish when they begin their first research project. The advantage of establishing a limited goal statement for your search is that once you have found your progenitor, you have reached a goal. You have accomplished something significant. Then, if you want to extend your search into the country of your ancestors' homeland you are free to establish a new goal.

Family history research has no obvious end or conclusion. If you allow it to take over, it will never end. For the sake of your own satisfaction and to derive a sense of accomplishment you must establish an end point, organize the information you have gathered, and make it available to other family members in written format. If you don't do that, when you die you will leave a filing cabinet overflowing with family history that will never see the light of day.

The following chart is intended to show you what a completed ancestors chart looks like. This chart was produced by a genealogy computer program. Pearl Ann Griffith is my mother.

 Feedback

Dear Jim,
Congratulations, you did a great job and have much to be proud of. The page on my dad was heart-warming for me. I was so young, just five, when he died. I have a lot of family history to digest here. Thank you and a big hug for this wonderful book.
Grace Kennedy

Actual Ancestors Chart

Ancestors of Pearl Ann Griffith

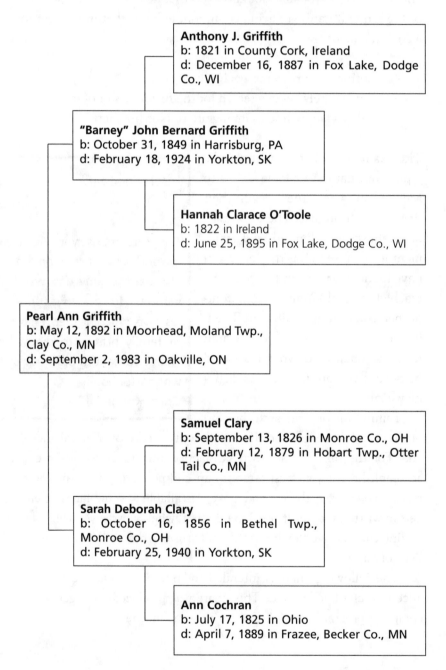

Anthony J. Griffith
b: 1821 in County Cork, Ireland
d: December 16, 1887 in Fox Lake, Dodge Co., WI

"Barney" John Bernard Griffith
b: October 31, 1849 in Harrisburg, PA
d: February 18, 1924 in Yorkton, SK

Hannah Clarace O'Toole
b: 1822 in Ireland
d: June 25, 1895 in Fox Lake, Dodge Co., WI

Pearl Ann Griffith
b: May 12, 1892 in Moorhead, Moland Twp., Clay Co., MN
d: September 2, 1983 in Oakville, ON

Samuel Clary
b: September 13, 1826 in Monroe Co., OH
d: February 12, 1879 in Hobart Twp., Otter Tail Co., MN

Sarah Deborah Clary
b: October 16, 1856 in Bethel Twp., Monroe Co., OH
d: February 25, 1940 in Yorkton, SK

Ann Cochran
b: July 17, 1825 in Ohio
d: April 7, 1889 in Frazee, Becker Co., MN

Family Group Sheets

The family group sheet (FGS) is the workhorse of family history. It is a form that shows information about one immediate family. This includes the husband, wife, and children. Children are numbered underneath the information about the husband and wife. While family group sheets vary in design, they essentially call for the same information: full names, date and place of birth, date and place of marriage, date and place of death, and so forth. On your parents' FGS you will be shown as a child. If you marry and have children, you and your wife will head a new FGS on which your children will also appear. The process repeats itself for each new generation. *See the completed FGS for my grandparents that follows.*

Later on we will discuss what information to look for and how to record it. Most of the facts you gather should be entered on the family group sheet. It won't be long before you have accumulated 100 or more family group sheets with information about your kin. Some sheets will be complete with information, while others will show numerous blank spaces waiting to be filled.

Throughout your research, use the family group sheets as your storehouse for information and your source of family reference.

If you intend to work by hand you will physically handle hundreds of family group sheets. If you use a genealogy computer program you will enter family information into the computer on what is called "the family card." Later you will print out family group sheets as you require them. The FGS is for storing information only, it is not intended to be placed in your completed book. As you will see later on, computer programs provide a much more attractive format for presenting family history to your readers.

Where to Get Blank Forms

- If you use a genealogy program you can print out blank family group sheets whenever you wish from your own program.

This is the first page of a family group sheet showing my grandparents and 3 of their 14 children.

Family Group Sheet

Husband	'Barney' John Bernard Griffith	
Born	31 Oct 1849	Harrisburg, PA[6]
Died	18 Feb 1924	Yorkton, SK
Buried	Feb 1924	Yorkton Municipal Cemetery
Alias	Barney	
Father	Anthony J. Griffith (1821-1887)	**Mother** Hannah Clarace O'Toole (1822-1895)
Married	30 Oct 1873	Hobart, Otter Tail Co., MN[8]

Wife	**Sarah Deborah Clary**	
Born	16 Oct 1856	Bethel Twp., Monroe Co., OH
Died	25 Feb 1940	Yorkton, SK
Buried		Yorkton Municipal Cem.
Father	Samuel Clary (1826-1879)	**Mother** Ann Cochran (1825-1889)

Children

1	M	Anthony 'Tony' Samuel[3] Griffith	
	Born	13 Sep 1874	Perham, Otter Tail Co., MN[3]
	Died	6 Jun 1941	Willowbrook, SK
	Alias	Tony	
	Spouse	Annie Elizabeth Rattray	
	Married	3 Apr 1901	

2	M	'Elmer' Frank Edmond Griffith	
	Born	1 Feb 1877	Frazee, MN
	Baptism	19 May 1877	Perham, Otter Tail Co., MN
	Died	25 Feb 1923	Rock Dell, SK
	Buried		Rock Dell Cemetery, SK
	Spouse	Maria 'Georgeanna' Celima D'Aoust	
	Married	8 Sep 1908	Yorkton, SK

3	M	John Bernard Griffith	
	Born	11 Apr 1878	Luce, (near Perham) Otter Tail Co., MN
	Baptism	14 Apr 1878	Perham, Otter Tail Co., MN
	Died	15 Mar 1963	Saskatoon, SK
	Buried	18 Mar 1963	Woodlawn Cemetery Saskatoon, SK
	Spouse	Julia Selina Sullivan	
	Married	6 Jun 1905	Cherryfield, SK

4	F	Hattie Griffith	
	Born	15 May 1879	Perham, Otter Tail Co., MN
	Died	5 Sep 1879	Perham, Otter Tail Co., MN[2]
	Buried		St. Henry Cem., Perham, MN

5	F	Emma Agnes Griffith	
	Born	4 Jun 1880	Perham, Otter Tail Co., MN
	Baptism	23 Jun 1880	Perham, Otter Tail Co., MN
	Died	29 Dec 1880	Perham, Otter Tail Co., MN

6	F	Sarah Griffith	
	Born	20 Sep 1881	Perham, Otter Tail Co., MN
	Died	27 Dec 1965	Saskatoon, SK
	Buried		Marengo, SK
	Spouse	John 'Jack' Sullivan	
	Married	10 Jun 1903	Cherryfield, SK

7	M	Charles Griffith	
	Born	3 Mar 1883	Perham, Otter Tail Co., MN
	Died	27 Jan 1948	Winnipeg, MB
	Spouse	Katherine 'Katie' Sullivan	
	Married	3 Jun 1908	Yorkton, SK

- If you are recording all information by hand there are several places you can obtain blank FGS sheets: approach your local library for assistance, ask your local genealogy society, ask a friend with a genealogy computer program to print out a blank form, then make copies.

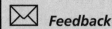 **Feedback**

Dear Jim,
It will be nice for our sons, their families, and future generations to know about their ancestors. You can feel proud of a job well done.
Ted & Pat Alberts

- Go to the *Family Tree* Magazine Web site, then click on Tool Kit, and you will be presented with an array of blank genealogy charts and forms you can download for free. The site is: http://www.familytreemagazine.com.
- Ancestry.com also offers various forms. Go to: http://www.ancestry.com/save/charts/ancchart.htm

Always Work Backwards

One of the basic rules of family history research is to move from the known to the unknown. That means going backwards in time, always proving a direct family linkage between each "older" generation. Start with yourself and your immediate family. Once you find your grandfather, search for his parents and so forth.

Send a blank family group sheet to your kinfolk with a covering letter asking them to make more blank copies, complete the FGS sheets for each of their families, and return the completed sheets to you.

The data required on the FGS is obvious, but you want more than that. Eventually, you want to assemble your material into an interesting family history format that you can present to your extended family. Now is the time to begin gathering the information that will allow you to prepare that exciting family history. Therefore, in addition to requesting a completed family group sheet, ask for such items as:

- Old letters,
- Newspaper clippings,
- Documents and certificates,
- Obituaries,
- Diaries,
- Copies of entries in family bibles,
- Old and current family photographs,
- Stories or articles that may have appeared in publications such as school or church centennial booklets, or
- Names of towns to accompany the birth, marriage, and death dates.

When asking for family data you should emphasize that you want the maiden name of a man's wife. John Ogilvy married Mary Jones, and that's the name you want on the FGS, not Mary Ogilvy.

Gain Their Trust

When you request such items as photographs and old documents, your covering letter must provide assurance that you will return them promptly. Then, when people begin sending you their treasured pictures and documents, you must make the necessary copies and return the material in good condition without delay. If you don't, word will spread like wildfire and your mailbox will be forever empty. I made it a rule to return pictures and documents within one week.

When you write to your relatives ask for their help with current addresses of kinfolk you have been unable to reach. If you have several glaring holes in your ancestors chart, ask your relatives if they can provide you with clues as to where they may be living or where you may be able to find information about them.

 Feedback

Dear Jim,
Many thanks for an excellent job of putting the Griffith family history together.
Bettie Alberts

Sources of Information

There are numerous sources to search out for information about your ancestors. Oftentimes you find yourself at a dead end, but every once in a while you hit pay dirt, and that's what keeps you going. Here's a listing of sources to keep in mind:

- Cemeteries
- Censuses
- Church histories
- Courthouses for wills, deeds etc.
- Family bibles
- Federal and Provincial Archives
- Historical societies
- Church of Jesus Christ of Latter-day Saints (Mormon Church)
- Libraries
- Military records
- Municipality yearbooks and histories
- Parish registers
- Personal interviews
- School records and histories
- Ships passenger lists
- Tax records
- The Internet
- Your relatives

Note: Do not buy generic family histories; they are worthless.

How to Get the Information

Knowing where to go for information and actually getting the information you want are two different things. Here are a few suggestions that will make your task easier and more productive.

 Feedback

Dear Jim,
Thank you for a wonderful addition to my library. It was a great idea to put in all those photos, it makes the book so much more interesting. What a tremendous amount of research you had to do. And the way you coordinated all that information. I find it amazing.
Margaret & Doug Sleeth

1. Get Up to Speed

If it's worth doing, it's worth doing well, so why not learn as much as you can about genealogy. Here are some ideas:

- Take a course in genealogy. Your local library will be able to give you assistance.
- Join a genealogy society in your area.
- Read books on family history.
- Explore the Internet.
- Visit the Church of Jesus Christ of Latter-day Saints family history centre.
- Talk to others about their research experience.

2. Create Template Paragraphs

Gathering information means that you will be making requests for data from a variety of sources. In the course of your search you will write a lot of letters, so try to reduce the amount of time you spend on each letter. Since certain parts of each letter will repeat the same information, prepare a few "template paragraphs" you can insert into your letters. This will save you considerable time and frustration.

 Feedback

Dear Jim,
Congratulations. We received your Griffith book and are enjoying it immensely. At last, we are able to tell our children "where we came from."
Adeline Pekar

3. Use the Phone

Half of your search time is spent waiting for people to reply to correspondence, so it's a good idea to use the phone more often. These days, when you can make a long-distance call for the price of a couple of postage stamps it makes sense to use the phone. This applies to government offices as well as relatives. I found that when I phoned a relative I didn't know and explained where I fit into the family it removed potential barriers and set the stage for a more fruitful response to my written requests for information.

4. Go E-mail

If you have a computer and are on the Internet, make good use of it. Get as many of your relatives' e-mail addresses as you can, for corresponding by e-mail will speed up your response time. It's a good idea to include your e-mail address on all your regular correspondence so that people will know that you are on the Internet and initiate more e-mail correspondence.

5. Frequent Your Library

Make liberal use of the library. You will find a large section of how-to books on genealogy. With the advent of the computer and e-mail, how-to information has changed considerably, so focus on more recent and up-to-date books.

 Feedback

Dear Jim,
I'm very impressed with the Griffith book. I realize now what a lot of time, talent, and research it involved. It will mean a lot to the younger generation later on.
Valerie Griffith

6. The Old Way Is Okay

You don't need a computer to gather information, but it does help. I recently met a lady who proudly showed me three large binders full of self-designed family group sheets all completed by hand. She also had numerous photos and stories. So don't hold back because you don't have a computer — after all, computers weren't even around a few years ago.

7. Visit the Church of Jesus Christ of Latter-day Saints

The Church of Jesus Christ of Latter-day Saints, also known as the Mormon Church, has a huge family history library. Find out where these churches are located in your city and visit their centres. They could be your best source of information. The data is stored on micro-fiche and microfilm at their local family history centres. They have more than 3,400 family history centres in 75 countries, so there is like-ly one in your area. Housed at the Church's headquarters in Salt Lake City, Utah are more than 2 million rolls of microfilmed genealogical records, 742,000 microfiche records, and 300,000 books. They have more than 240 cameras currently microfilming in nearly 44 countries. Most of the records are earlier than 1920. You may conduct research at their family history centres by appointment, free of charge. There is, however, a small fee to bring in a microfilm from Salt Lake City.

8. About Census Records

Remember to search out Census returns, for they can yield consider-able useful data. Census returns contain the official enumeration of the Canadian population. For most provinces, the returns of 1851, 1861, 1871, 1881, 1891, and 1901 list each person individually, with details as to age, sex, country or province of birth, religion, racial or ethnic origin, occupation, marital status, and education. Census records are available at all major libraries.

 Feedback

Dear Jim,
Thanks again for the many hours you devoted to bringing our fam-ily history together for the benefit of all descendants.
Bernadine Harper

At present, the 1901 census is the last return available for public view-ing. Census returns subsequent to 1901 are closed under the Statistics Act, which contains strict confiden-tiality provisions that protect the information indefinitely.

To conduct a productive search of census records, you must know the approximate locality of your ances-tor, as the returns are arranged by township or parish within each county. Small towns and villages are enumerated within their respective townships; larger towns and cities are listed separately. For more information about Canada census records and links to many other government sites of interest to researchers, visit: www.archives.ca. You may also write: National Archives of Canada,

395 Wellington St., Ottawa, ON, K1A 0N3, or phone General Reference: 1-866-578-7777, Reference Services: 613-992-3884, or Genealogy Reference: 613-996-7458.

Computers Make It Easier

Computers have radically changed the way people conduct their family history research, how they record their findings, and how they prepare the family history for printing. Here's a closer look at each of these areas.

Genealogy Software

A genealogy software program provides you with an easy way to enter and store such family history information as names, dates, facts, and notes about each individual family member. Best of all, these programs automatically create genealogy reports, charts, and forms with each individual correctly linked to the appropriate family. As you may have surmised, accurate output is highly dependant upon accurate entries.

Several years ago there were only a few genealogy programs on the market, but today there are dozens. So which one should you buy, and what makes one better than the other? Some of the programs you may wish to check out are: Family Tree Maker, Generations Grande Suite, and Brother's Keeper. If you have a Macintosh, look into Reunion, a genealogy program made only for Macintosh computers.

All programs are not created equal. Here are some things you should ask about:

- Is it a stable program — does it perform the way it was intended to?
- Does the program contain flaws or bugs that have not been corrected for some time?
- Does the company provide good technical support? Is it easy to reach by e-mail or phone? Will tech support help you?

- Does the program have a good reference manual and on-line help?

Where possible, get a personal recommendation from satisfied users before making your purchase. You can find these people by checking with your local genealogy society or scouring the Internet and the Web site of the program you are investigating.

The following Web sites provide comprehensive information about genealogy software programs:

- http://genealogy.about.com/cs/genealogysoftware
  From this "About" site, click on Software for Windows or Software for Macintosh and you will be presented with a comprehensive list of genealogy software programs. Be sure to check out Family Tree Maker.
- http://www.cyndislist.com
  Cyndi's List is the most comprehensive genealogy site on the Internet. Click to her Software & Computers page (www.cyndislist.com/software.htm) to find system requirements, prices, ordering information, vendors' names and addresses, and program features for numerous software programs on the market.

Visit our Web site at www.after 50.ca, where you can find a list of great Web sites related to genealogy. From our home page, just click on "Resource Links," then "Active Mind," then "Ancestors."

Genealogy Training On-line

The Centre for Continuing Education at the University of Regina offers an eight-week on-line genealogy training course for adults 55 and older entitled "Tell Your Story." At the time of this writing the cost of the course is $65. Your computer screen is your classroom. There are weekly lessons and homework but no exams. What a great way to learn how to conduct family history research. Get in touch with the centre and find out more. Its Web site is at www.seniorcentre.ca/docs/studies/genealogy.html. Write to: Seniors' Education Centre, Centre for Continuing Education, University of Regina, Regina, SK, S4S 0A2. Ph.: 306-585-5722.

Has Your Surname Been Searched?

While conducting research for your family ancestors, be on the lookout for existing research that may have been completed for your family surname. Check the Internet for Web sites with your family name and for family history information from the area where your relatives once lived.

 Feedback

Dear Jim,

Congratulations on a job well done! We are thrilled with your book on the Griffith family. The additional background research is so interesting along with the family history. Our entire family, all the Griffiths and many generations to come will now know their roots. Thank you for the gift of knowledge you have passed on to all of us.

Heather & Louis Kolla

If you do find individual names or a family history with the same surname as yours, be sure to establish a verifiable linkage before including the names in your family tree.

Also investigate message boards and search sites devoted to identifying those who are searching for a particular surname. Lady Luck does strike once in a while. Several years ago while researching my grandmother, whose maiden name was Clary, I learned from the Wisconsin Archives Office that a lady in Michigan was researching the same Clary family. I contacted the lady in Michigan and learned that a complete family history of the Clarys had been written some years previously. As a result I was able to purchase one of the few remaining copies, and sure enough my grandmother and all her ancestors were recorded in that history of the Clarys.

There are various sites on the Internet where you can enter your surname and get a list of places where your surname has appeared. Who knows, you may get lucky. Try these:

- Roots Web will produce a list of places to go if you enter your surname. It also contains dozens of genealogy links. Go to:

http://www.rootsweb.com.

- Here's another site to help you in your surname search. It also has various family history links such as message board locations. Visit: http://www.familyhistory.com.
- Another family finder is: http://www.genealogy.com.

 Feedback

Dear Jim,
What a wonderful job you did on the Griffith book. It is a quality work.
Mary Laski

Visit the Places They Lived

Once you have gathered a significant amount of information about your immediate family and made a complete search of the Internet you might like to visit the places where your ancestors lived. Not only will it be a rewarding experience, but during your visit you are sure to unearth more information. While planning your visit to your ancestors' former communities you should be prepared to visit churches, cemeteries, newspaper offices, and other places where old records are kept. If there are relatives in the area you will want to visit them as well. Bring along whatever reference materials you will need and don't forget your camera. When looking at old tombstones you will find that over the years the engraving or lettering will appear washed out and difficult to read or photograph. To bring the lettering to life, rub it with a block of Styrofoam available at most craft stores. You will be amazed at the results.

During the time I researched my ancestors, Olga and I travelled to Wisconsin, Minnesota, P.E.I., Cape Breton, and Saskatchewan. Not only did we find the trips exciting and interesting, we met new people and gathered new material everywhere we went.

How to Organize Your Data

Over the years, as you gather family history information, the data you collect will begin to take up more and more space. Unless you have your material well organized, your correspondence and documents will become one big clutter of paper and you will find it difficult to locate anything without a major search.

Here are a few tips that will enable you to lay your fingers on anything you want within a few seconds.

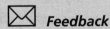 **Feedback**

Dear Jim,
What an amazing history of the Griffith family!
Pat & Nick Hertz

The following suggestions are based on the assumption that you have a computer and are using a genealogy program.

a) When you receive a completed handwritten FGS (family group sheet) from a relative, enter the data into your computer, print out a copy of the FGS, and place it under the right tab in the appropriate binder. Devise your own system for organizing your binders and the tabs within each binder. Consider organizing your binders by generation and by family.

b) When you receive materials from your relatives, scan or copy documents or snapshots and return appropriate material within one week.

c) Mark the handwritten FGS copy as "entered" (into the computer, that is), date it, and place it along with the covering letter and your response in the appropriate file folder.

d) If you asked for and received a picture of a relative and his family along with the FGS, make a photocopy of the picture and affix it to the FGS printout. There are two reasons for this step.

    1) When looking at the FGS you will know at a glance that you have a picture of that family in your computer.

2) If you don't personally know that relative you now have his or her picture affixed to his FGS and that will avoid any mix-up later on when preparing your family history book.

e) Most of the completed FGSs you receive from your relatives will actually be incomplete. As a result, when you send your response, it's a good idea to enclose a computer printout of their FGS and ask that they complete the missing items and return it.

Get It between the Covers

When you take on the task of researching your ancestors it is not your intention to hide your findings from others. Your plan is to share the results of your work with your relatives. One way to share is to organize your material into a book format and get a copy out to all your kinfolk.

What follows is a sequence of eight steps that will help you transform your research into beautifully bound books for your kin.

My discussion is based on the assumption that you are using a genealogy computer program. I also assume that you have been collecting pictures, stories, newspaper articles, obituaries, and other items of interest in addition to names and dates of family members. I have seen genealogies that consisted of nothing more than names and dates, without a word of where the people lived or whether they made a living as a farmer, a storekeeper, or a blacksmith. Don't let that happen to your history; gather personal information about your ancestors and the period in which they lived. It's more work, but your book will be more interesting.

1. Establish a Stop Date

If you haven't already done so, establish a date or event at which time research stops, and it becomes time to (self) publish. If you don't, your research can go on forever.

2. Present Oldest to Youngest

In your book, present your research findings in a sequence that is the exact reverse of the way you collected it. In other words your oldest known ancestor is presented first, then his descendants and so forth down the line toward present-day generations. Actually, your computer program will look after that.

3. Generations Become Chapters

Think of your ancestors in terms of the generation they belong to. Your oldest known ancestor, possibly the original immigrant, will belong to the first generation, his children will be second generation, and so forth. On my mother's side I am a fourth-generation North American. On my father's side I am a sixth-generation Canadian.

 Feedback

Dear Jim,
I commend you on the wonderful job you have done in researching the family and organizing this valuable history. I have never come across a family history so well put together. I was most impressed by the additional information you included on each and every family member. The pictures, homestead documents, letters, etc. add to the richness of this volume. Thank you for providing us with this rich and colourful history.
Bill Tonita

To make it easy for the reader to stay oriented, make each generation a chapter. Therefore your Chapter 1 will contain your first generation ancestors. Chapter 2 will contain your second generation ancestors, and so forth. By taking that approach, all of your uncles and aunts will be in the same chapter, and all of your brothers and sisters will be in the same chapter. Most computer programs will also divide printouts by generation.

4. Do a Last-Chance Check

You don't want to go to press with your book until you feel confident that your information is accurate and complete. The best way to do a final check is go back to the source. Run off what is called a descendants report (shown below) for each major family and send it to a couple of responsible relatives in each family group. Ask them to carefully check it for missing items as well as spelling of names, dates, etc. I guarantee they will find errors or omissions in your data. As you can see from the descendants report below, it permits you to crowd a lot of information onto a page. Each software program will produce a slightly different style of report but the basics are the same.

A Partial Descendants Report

1. Samuel CLARY (1786–) & Cordelia HARRISON (1791–)
    1. Enoch CLARY (1811–1891) & Asneath HARVEY (1817–1879)
        1. Lucinda CLARY (1836–) & Thomas V. RHINE
        2. William CLARY (1838–) & Elizabeth ? (1843–)
        3. Elizabeth Ann CLARY (1842–1868) & John A. DOUGLAS
        4. Lydia CLARY (1844–) & Samuel MILLER
    2. Samuel CLARY (1826–1879) & Ann COCHRAN (1825–1889)
        1. Martin Van Buren CLARY (1848–1923) & Susan McNULTY (1858–1905)
        2. Cordelia A. CLARY (1852–)
        3. John Daniel CLARY (1853–1927) & Mary DURKAN (1861–1921)
        4. Sarah Deborah CLARY (1856–1940) & "Barney" John GRIFFITH (1849–1924)

5. Do a Practice Run

For various reasons, you must produce a sample copy of your book complete with Introduction, Table of Contents, and Index. Here are some of the reasons you need this draft copy:
- to get an estimate of the number of pages in the book,
- to show two or more printers so they can give you a printing quote, and
- to analyze it for ways to make improvements.

6. Observations about Format

Most computer programs will give you a choice of report styles. I prefer what is called the register report. It automatically creates a narrative paragraph for each individual, beginning with the couple of your choice, and then includes all of their descendants. Each descendant is assigned a number, beginning with 1 for the source person. The entire report in also divided into generations and an index is included at the end. Following is a sample register report for Anthony J. Griffith.

*Note: **Do not** include family group sheets in your book; they are designed for gathering information only. **Please do** include descendants charts at appropriate locations in your book. The chart will make it easier for the reader to follow the family history and know where he or she fits in to the big picture.*

A Sample Register Report

1. **Anthony J. GRIFFITH** was born 1821 in County Cork, Ireland. Anthony died 16 Dec 1887 in Fox Lake, Dodge Co., Wisconsin, at the age of 67, and was buried in St. Mary's Catholic Cemetery, Fox Lake, WI. Occupation: Farmer. Residence: Fox Lake and Westford, Dodge Co., WI. Religion: Roman Catholic. He married Hannah Clarace O'TOOLE about 1842 in Ireland. She was born 1822 in Ireland. Hannah died 25 Jun 1895 in Fox Lake, Dodge County, Wisconsin, at the age of 73, and was buried in St. Mary's Catholic Cemetery, Fox Lake, WI.

They had 10 children:

2.	m	i.	Michael A. GRIFFITH	b. 1843
3.	m	ii.	Charles GRIFFITH	b. 1845
4.	f	iii.	Mary GRIFFITH	b. 1847
5.	m	iv.	"Barney" John Bernard GRIFFITH	b. 31 Oct 1849 d. 18 Feb 1924
6.	f	v.	Jane "Jennie" GRIFFITH	b. 1852
7.	f	vi.	Catherine GRIFFITH	b. 1856
8.	m	vii.	George W. GRIFFITH	b. 1857

9.	m	viii.	Anthony GRIFFITH	b. Nov 1859	
10.	f	ix.	Agnes "Hannah" L. GRIFFITH	b. 1863	d. 16 May 1901
11.	m	x.	William H. GRIFFITH	b. 30 Jul 1866	d. 11 Feb 1940

Immediately below the list of children, include whatever narrative you may have regarding the parents of the family. I began as shown in the excerpt below:

When Anthony and Hannah left Ireland in 1848 the Potato Famine was at its peak. It is generally accepted that the Great Famine lasted for six years, from 1845 to 1851. We will probably never know for certain why our ancestors choose to leave when they did, but ...

7. Get Price Quotes

You need price quotes for the following items:

- Printing the book.
- Binding the book. You will have to seek out a book binder who binds small quantities of about 200 books. You will also have to decide on hard cover or soft cover.
- Cover design. You may be able to do this yourself.
- Mailing cost. Take your sample book to the post office. Weigh it and arrive at an average cost of mailing to your relatives.
- Other: you may have other production costs related to your book.

Once you have all this information put together you have a price to quote your relatives when you write them to find out how many books they want to order.

8. Sales Pitch to Your Relatives

In many respects this letter to your relatives is a sales pitch. They have no idea what your book will look like so you have to tell them. If you think it's going be a top-notch book, tell your relatives what a great book you have. Keep your letter to one page. Although it will be a "form" letter, personalize it with a greeting such as "Dear Jack and Betty." Here are the highlights of what to include in your letter:

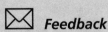 **Feedback**

Dear Jim,

The Griffith book is very interesting and I can see it was a terrific amount of work. Thank you for writing it. It is indeed a keepsake.

Marjorie Alberts

- Describe your book: number of pages, pictures, charts, type of binding, type of cover, stories, how many individuals, and whatever else is special about it.

- Tell them the price of a book. Advise that the price represents printing, binding, and mailing costs only. Don't expect to get reimbursed for your time or the out-of-pocket expenses you incurred over the years.

- If corresponding with American relatives, quote in U.S. funds.

- Advise that the number of books you get printed will be based on how many orders you receive from them. Stress that this is the time to order their book(s).

- Set a time limit for receipt of book orders. Six weeks after date of letter is fair.

- Ask that they enclose a cheque to cover the cost of books ordered. Always get the money first to save potential problems later on. For the same reason, it's a good idea to make a photocopy of cheques received and keep a record of books ordered and paid for as well as date of shipment.

- Give them your best estimate of when the books will be ready to mail.

When the time comes to place your order with the printer, order 15 to 20 percent more books than you received orders for. Invariably some of your relatives will want to order additional books and some who neglected to order will change their minds and want one or more copies.

Take a Break

While you wait for book orders to arrive from your relatives, take a well-deserved break from genealogy work and get away for while. A few weeks later you will be back into the swing of things as you attend to printing, binding, and packaging your books ready for mailing. Just before wrapping a book take a moment to personalize your work by signing and dating one of the front pages.

QUICK SUMMARY

- Family history research is a rewarding experience. If you are interested, start now. It's never too late.

- Make use of the tools available, such as ancestor charts, family group sheets, and descendants reports.

- A genealogy software program is a great help in organizing your data and printing out reports.

- Lean heavily on your relatives for information; that's where the family history resides.

- Establish a completion time, get your data into book format and out to your kinfolk as soon as possible.

In this chapter:

- Follow the prompts, think a while, and identify your learning interests.

- Find out about adult learning opportunities at universities and colleges.

- Discover the advantages of distance learning — it may be right for you.

Education is a journey not a destination.

The Sky's the Limit

If you have any doubts about the relevance of this chapter to the 50-plus age group, pause for a moment and ask yourself, "How many adults do I know who are presently engaged in some type of learning activity?" The odds are that you know of at least two or three who are exercising their mind part-time.

Four people in my extended family spring to mind as being mentally active in a learning environment: one is studying for a university degree, one is upgrading his computer skills, one is taking an English course, and one is attending a series of university lectures. And they are all seniors! So what's going on — why all this interest in learning?

The answer is simple enough: all of these learners want something. While it may not be down on paper, they all have a goal, they want to achieve something. For some, it is learning for the sake of learning. Their newly acquired knowledge will provide them with tremendous satisfaction and personal fulfillment. For others the goal may be more tangible and fill a practical need. As a consequence of what they learned, they will be able to do something they were unable to do before.

Whether your goal is to acquire a little more wisdom in your old age, learn how to navigate the Web, or learn how to frame a picture, I say well done, keep it up.

The purpose of this chapter is to add another category to your repertoire of ways to satisfy your hungry mind. As you will soon see, in this chapter we explore a wide selection of learning opportunities, ranging from acquiring a university degree via distance education to learning the strategies of smart investing. As alluded to in previous chapters, if you have time on your hands there is no reason to sit idle allowing your mind and body to wither away. Wherever you live, there are endless ways to maintain an active mind. We'll show you a few, but the sky is the limit.

Follow Your Dreams

Most people have a book of dreams. You will find yours tucked away in a private corner or your mind where only you have right of entry. It's a very special place that you access every once in a while. You gaze at your book of dreams for a while, then return it for safe keeping until next time.

Take a moment now to open your dream book. In your mind, flip through the pages and see what you have entered over the years. When you come to the entries about finding prince charming or winning the lottery, pass them by, for we can't help you there. Keep looking, find your pages about "learning." What sort of knowledge have you yearned for over the years but never had the time or the inclination to pursue?

Could it be that you have always wanted to study astronomy, geography, or political science, but never found time? When you were younger, did you begin a course of study but leave it uncompleted? Now that you have more time you may want to revisit that area of study and finish it off.

Maybe a set of unfortunate circumstances prevented you from completing high school. If over the years your dream book reflects a lingering desire to get your high school certificate, it can be done.

Now that your working years are drawing to a close you will have a new outlook on life and a new set of priorities. From your new perspective you may have renewed interest in such things as Canadian studies, writing, or learning to play a musical instrument.

Let's not forget the fun stuff. If you have always wanted to be a belly dancer or an actor but never had the time or the daring to take that plunge, this may be your opportunity.

This is your very own dream book. If you decide to get involved in a learning activity, be sure to follow your own dreams and not someone else's. Establish your own personal goals for your own reasons and take it from there. Whatever learning you decide to focus upon at this stage in your life, it should be enjoyable, certainly not a daily grind or a chore.

ACTIVITY # 9:

Get it down on paper before you lose the thought. What are your learning interests? In the space below jot down the learning interest you would like to pursue.

What are your learning interests?

Adults Eager to Learn

Here's some interesting information based on Statistics Canada's Profile of Adult Learners. It appears that learning has become a life-long process for many Canadians.

- Every year, about 6 million adult Canadians participate in education and training activities. That's about one in four adult Canadians.
- Men and women are equally likely to take part in some form of learning.
- Those between 25 and 44 years of age are more likely to take part in learning — about 37 percent engage in learning activities.
- Only 10 percent of those 55 and older are likely to take part in learning activities, but that number is growing.
- About 57 percent of adult learners get involved in learning activities for job or career reasons, 29 percent for personal interest, and 14 percent for both.
- The percentage of lifelong learners increases from east to west across Canada. At 35 percent, British Columbians are most likely to pursue adult learning, while those in Newfoundland are the least likely at 19 percent.

Journey of Learning

When I first noticed Marlane's article in *The Booster*, I knew that her sincere message belonged in the learning chapter of this book. Thanks Marlane for sharing it with out readers.

Going back to school can open your mind and satiate your spirit
by Marlane Tibbs

Ten years ago I signed on for an extended expedition that will shortly be coming to a close.

Barring complications, I expect to have my final papers approved and certified and will most probably return to a more settled life in May. Overall, my journey has been a complete success, but I am now beginning to feel the need for rest and reflection.

By now, those of you who know me must be thinking I've been into the herbal teas again. Really, I'm quite sober ... the expedition I'm referring to is the 10 years I've spent as a part-time mature student in the quest for my degree at the University of Toronto at Mississauga, as it is now called. This May I will graduate with a major in religious studies and a minor in literature. It has been both an adventure and a privilege to have taken this journey. Let me share some of the insights I have picked up along the way.

The most important point I would like to share is that education is the most priceless gift you will ever receive this side of heaven. I feel I can make this statement with certainty since I have taken courses to complete my high school diploma, courses just for fun at night school, practical courses in community college, and finally, I have completed a BA at the university level. We are so fortunate to live in Mississauga, where education has been made available to meet the diverse needs of our multicultural, multi-faceted community.

Having said this, I'd like to clear up a few misconceptions about going back to school. These are the five reasons I most often hear from people who would like to go back to school but think they can't because: education is too expensive, they have a family, they're working, they feel they are not smart enough, or they are too old.

Of course, these are all valid reasons to a point. However, the old adage "Where there is a will, there is a way" provides a powerful counterpoint to these concerns. It has been my experience that once you set your sights on a goal and decide to go for it, many avenues suddenly open up which you might not have previously known existed. I have had the great good fortune to have met men and women of just about every age and ethnic background imaginable. Their circumstances have been varied, but they have all had one goal in mind — they have wanted to improve themselves, to maximize their potential.

Single moms go back to school because they want a better life for themselves and their children. They refuse to be condemned to a miserable minimum wage existence. Stay-at-home moms (like me) who have raised their children finally feel free to pursue a career. Dads are no exception. They are out there upgrading their skills or their level of education to make themselves a more valuable employee.

Interestingly enough, most parents I have talked to have very close, supportive families. Their children more willingly do chores because they are proud of their parents' accomplishments. They understand that they are helping to contribute in a very real way to a better life in the future. (However, I found out that they don't necessarily want to hear about what went on in forensics class at the dinner table!)

Of course, lots of people take courses just for fun and to meet like-minded people. As far as age goes, I know two very mature students at U of T, one in her 80s and one in his 70s. Both take courses just to keep their minds active.

If you do decide to go back to school, particularly if you are goal-oriented and plan to upgrade yourself, expect to work hard. Be disciplined and determined. Take a positive attitude and meet the challenges with an open mind. Expect to hit bumps and curves along the way. If you knew everything to begin with, you wouldn't need to be there. With the right approach, education can be a thrilling ride.

What's your destination?

Where to Find Education

Numerous educational institutions across the country are in the business of dispensing knowledge. Whatever your interests, you are sure to find a course of study to fit your needs. There are more than 150 universities and colleges in Canada with every province and territory represented. Here are three quick ways to find out where they are located and obtain detailed information about each one of them.

- The Internet: Here are two Web sites listing universities and colleges in Canada. From these sites you can click your way to the Web site for each individual university or college:

  http://www.campusaccess.com
  http://www.uwaterloo.ca/canu

- Your local library: Always a great resource, your local library will have directories of Canadian colleges and universities, as well as continuing education course catalogues for local institutions.
- *Maclean's* Magazine: In a special annual "Guide to Canadian Universities & Colleges," *Maclean's* profiles, ranks, and provides comprehensive data about universities and colleges in Canada. If the current guide is no longer available on the newsstands, you will be able to review a copy at your local library.

Choices at a University

As a 50-plus reader, you should focus on the department of continuing education and what it has to offer at the university of your choice. This department provides educational opportunities for part-time, mature, and evening students. Here's an overview of what it offers:

- A wide variety of degree programs;
- Thousands of courses, seminars, and workshops on a diverse range of subject areas;
- Many offer a series of lectures on interesting topics and there are no exams to write; and
- You can often elect to attend university on campus or take your course by distance learning over the Internet. More on this later in the chapter.

If you are interested, pick up the phone and order a catalogue from the university of your choice or search its Web site for more detailed information.

Choices at a Community College

Community college courses tend to reflect the essential skills needed in today's workplace. Most colleges offer programs in the highest growth occupations, from computer programming to health studies, science, and financial management. At a community college you can:

- Enroll in a wide variety of certificate or diploma programs;
- Become a part-time student selecting one or more subjects from a wide range of non-credit courses; and
- Enroll in courses that are offered on-line in the distance learning format.

Just recently Centennial College in Toronto did a profile of its students. One of their findings was that 12 percent of their part-time students were 45 years of age or older. While the 45-plus age category does not quite match our target audience of 50-plus, it makes the point that a sizeable portion of part-time college students are middle age. If you feel that a college will provide the course you want, order its catalogue or search its Web site for detailed information.

A Consortium of Ontario Colleges

OntarioLearn.com is a consortium of 22 Ontario community colleges that have partnered to develop and deliver over 290 on-line courses. Each partner college selects courses from the OntarioLearn.com course inventory that will complement its existing distance education offerings. This partnership approach has allowed member colleges to avoid duplication and, more importantly, increase the availability of on-line learning opportunities for their students.

Through this virtual classroom environment, students can pursue their educational goals, whether they be the completion of a single course or the fulfillment of a college certificate or diploma. Students can take courses from their home or office, accessing the courses at their convenience. Course instructors and fellow classmates may live anywhere in Canada or somewhere else in the world. The OntarioLearn Web site can be found at www.ontariolearn.com. Within this Web site you can find a list of the 22 colleges in the partnership along with their phone numbers and Web sites.

Canadian Education on the Web

The Web site www.oise.utoronto.ca/~mpress/eduweb brings together everything relating to Canada and education that has a presence on the World Wide Web. The page is developed and maintained by Marian Press within the Ontario Institute for Studies in Education. Here is a sample of the amazing lists contained on this site. If you want information about the Labrador School Board or the Coutts Library in Alberta, it's there, along with much more:

- Boards of education
- Commercial education sites
- Distance education
- Educators and education resources
- Independent institutions
- Ministries of education
- Private school organizations
- Provincial organizations
- Students' organizations
- Teachers' organizations
- Universities and colleges

A Small Sampling

Whatever course of study you are interested in you should be able to find it at a university or college in your area. In this chapter we aim to give you the tools and information that will make it easier for you to find what you are looking for at a university or college of your choice. With more than 150 universities and colleges to choose from we can focus on only a small number as we attempt to give you a picture of what's available.

Ryerson University Attracts the Over-50 Crowd

Along with the usual degree courses, certificate programs, and distance learning, Ryerson University in Toronto has a wide range of learning opportunities designed for the 50-plus population. Visit Ryerson's Web site at www.ryerson.ca.

Ryerson's SeniorCentre.ca offers seniors free on-line courses with titles such as Old Age Isn't For Sissies, Memoir Writing, and Internet Navigation. Visit: www.seniorcentre.ca.

The L.I.F.E. Institute offers older adults a wide range of courses and programs designed to provide opportunities for self-development and enrichment. There is a nominal membership fee, and study groups and instructor-led courses are charged on an individual basis. Contact the L.I.F.E. Institute at 416-979-5000 ext. 6989 or visit the Web site at www.ryerson.ca/~lifeinst.

Act II Studio is a theatre school where older adults have an opportunity to study the theatre and acting at every level. To learn more, phone 416-979-5000 ext. 6297 or visit www.ryerson.ca/~act2.

From the University of Toronto

The University of Toronto's School of Continuing Studies offers university-level courses and certification programs, in both evening and daytime classes. Its programs include such topics as arts, humanities, sciences, creative writing, professional writing, and English as a second language. Many of the courses are offered at a reduced fee to those over 55. The school also provides distance learning and on-line learning to thousands of students all over Ontario — and the world. Visit its Web site at http://learn.utoronto.ca.

Simon Fraser University, Burnaby, B.C.

The following welcome from Dr. Alan David Aberbach, program director for Simon Fraser, caught my eye as a most sincere invitation for seniors to take part in its educational programs. He is referring to non-credit courses in its fall program.

> As the Seniors Program begins its twenty-seventh year of service to the Greater Vancouver community, I am delighted to invite you to join us for our finest and most intellectually stimulating program of courses to date.
>
> Responding to numerous requests and to make it easier and more mentally stimulating for you, we have expanded each class session from two hours to two and one-half hours, and courses are now scheduled for every morning and early afternoon, six days a week.

The Opsimath Club at Simon Fraser sponsors a series of afternoon lectures on timely subjects. (An opsimath is someone who continues to learn late in life.) These free public lectures are open to all seniors and are followed by a discussion and/or debate.

University of Regina, Centre for Continuing Education

The Seniors' Education Centre is a partnership between the Seniors' University Group Inc. and the Centre for Continuing Education. Founded in 1977, it provides more than 100 older adult education programs in Regina and a variety of learning opportunities for seniors (age 55 and over) in several rural communities.

Tuition fees will be waived for seniors for most courses. Phone: 306-585-5816, or visit the Web site at www.uregina.ca/cce/seniors.

Canadian Virtual University

The Canadian Virtual University (CVU) is a partnership of 13 Canadian universities working together to offer complete university degrees or certificates on-line and through distance education. This is a great Web site providing instant information on what courses are available and where. Visit CVU at www.cvu-uvc.ca.

Tuition Fees for Seniors

Many universities offer a tuition fee reduction to seniors. Here is a sampling of what you may find.

- **University of Waterloo** offers a bursary equivalent to the tuition fee to all students 65 years and over who register for degree courses. See its catalogue for further details.
- **Laurentian University** waives tuition fees for Canadian citizens 60 years of age and over who enroll in university credit courses. They are, however, responsible for other fees outlined in the catalogue.
- **Lakehead University** offers half-price tuition and no activity fees to Canadian citizens who are 60 years of age and over who enroll in credit courses.
- **Athabasca University** offers Canadian citizens 65 years of age or over a reduction in course registration fees. Seniors pay the full course materials and handling fee portion of registration but are given a reduction of one-half the tuition registration fee. See its catalogue for more details.

Is Distance Learning Right for You?

The University of Waterloo began its distance education program in 1968 with the introduction of audio-taped physics courses. Today it offers about 175 courses.

Distance education is not a flash in the pan. Daniel Granger, director of distance education at the University of Minnesota, says, "We'll have more of it, and we'll have it in more shapes and sizes." Rich Halberg, director of California's Virtual University, adds, "The growth rate is astronomical." A spokesperson for an Ontario community college told me that enrolment in on-line courses has been increasing ten-fold each year.

Some institutions will allow you to sample part of an on-line course for a brief period of time. Try to get all the details you can about the kind of interaction you can expect before making your final decision.

Whether or not distance education is for you will depend on your individual situation and preferences. Here are some points to consider:

- If you live some distance from a university or college location, distance learning will enable you to access a learning opportunity without concern for commuting to a campus.
- Distance education allows you to have a flexible study schedule, but you must be able to study independently, manage your time well, and meet deadlines that you set for yourself.
- If you are motivated, have self-discipline and good reading and writing skills, distance learning may be for you.
- As a rule of thumb, expect to spend 10 hours a week for each course taken.

Computer Requirements

If you consider taking an on-line (distance learning) course of study, the university or college offering the course will advise you of the computer requirements. As a minimum, you will require a computer, a monitor, a connection to the Internet, a browser (Netscape or Internet Explorer), a personal e-mail account, a recent version of MS Word (or other word processor), a processor of adequate speed, and adequate RAM and hard disk drive space.

Study Tips

- Establish a study routine.
- Decide where you are going to study.

- Decide the time of day you are going to study. Most of us are most alert at certain times of the day; select that period as study time.
- Don't let others interrupt you during these times.

A Satisfying Experience

Helen, a friend from my home province of Saskatchewan, is feeling a lot more fulfilled these days. Thanks for sharing your thoughts, Helen. They may encourage others to fill the void in their lives.

I Knew I Was Capable of More
by Helen Nerby

When I retired in the early nineties I greeted the thought with enthusiasm. We would be free to set our own pace without obligation to the clock or the job. I was soon involved in two service clubs, the church, three bridge clubs, and always available to serve on whatever committee needed help. Eventually, I grew weary of the constant meetings and ongoing activities they created. I gradually withdrew and resigned from memberships. But what should I do instead?

As a teenager I foolishly left school in Grade 11 to work in an office. Later on I completed high school, but I have always felt that I had not acquired as much education as I am capable of.

One day, the subject came up in conversation with my brother. He encouraged and challenged me to pursue the educational goal. As we discussed the merits of further education, I realized that this was the route I wanted to take. But there were barriers. I would have to attend classes at the University of Regina, a two-hour return drive from Indian Head, not always possible in winter. And to satisfy my whim, no matter how commendable, the cost would be prohibitive. I kept the idea simmering in the back of my mind but never pursued it in any concrete way. Then fate stepped in to give me the nudge I needed.

I noticed an ad from the University of Waterloo. It offered distance education classes whereby the tuition was waived for "mature students" through a bursary. As a very mature student in my early 70s, my application was accepted without proof of previous academic enrolment.

I have now completed seven classes toward my BA. Since I don't have the computer capability to take my courses on-line, I maintain contact by telephone, regular mail, and e-mail. Course material may include taped lectures, notes, and the appropriate texts. Although I have not met any of the staff or professors in person, they are always ready to offer encouragement and assistance.

More than ever I am determined to obtain my degree about 2006 and accept my diploma in person in Waterloo! This project has challenged me, but it has also filled a large void. My studies have given me increased confidence, my enthusiasm is boundless, and I have learned that age is not an impediment to learning. I should have done it years ago!

Courses in Your Own Community

Here is a great way to keep your mind active and enjoy yourself at the same time. In most communities a centre for education and training works with your district school board to offer a variety of courses. They publish a catalogue of their courses, which will usually include computer courses, ESL classes, English and math upgrading, culinary arts, and business skills. Call your local city hall or school board for information. Some of the courses will sound like this:

- **Smart Investing** (8 evening sessions)
  Learn the financial strategies you need. Establish a sound plan and select good institutions for stocks, bonds, RRSPs, RRIFs, and other financial products.
- **Writing Better English** (8 evening sessions)
  Would you like to be able to write better ordinary, everyday English? The course will include basic grammar and spelling but will focus on improved sentence structure and composition.

Want to Finish High School?

If for one reason or another you didn't complete high school many years ago, you can do it now. Find out how many credits you need, select the subjects you find most interesting, and get started. If you live in Ontario and opt for the government correspondence course it's virtually free. First you pay a nominal fee, and then, if you meet certain requirements such as passing the course, your money is refunded.

Check out "Provincial Education" in your phone book and make a few phone calls about secondary education in your province. Procedures for getting your missing credits in Ontario are highlighted below. Your own province will have similar procedures.

You can also get your high school equivalency certificate by attending any school offering high school equivalency courses. But there are two drawbacks. First, you have to physically attend classroom courses, and second, there will be a fee in the range of $450. Seniors may be eligible for a discount.

Distance Education for Secondary Education in Ontario

As part of the Ontario Ministry of Education, the Independent Learning Centre (ILC) provides a wide range of distance education courses that allow adults (mature students) to earn secondary school diploma credits, upgrade their basic skills, or study for personal development. The Independent Learning Centre offers two kinds of correspondence courses:

- secondary school credit courses leading to an Ontario secondary school diploma, and
- non-credit adult basic education courses in adult basic literacy, English as a second language (ESL), and courses for upgrading in English and mathematics.

The credits you earn are the same as those earned at any secondary school in Ontario. Every ILC course meets the requirements of the

Ontario Ministry of Education. Your success with ILC courses depends on your motivation and persistence. Because there are no classes, you will have to rely on your own work habits and eagerness to learn. However, you will not be totally alone. Qualified teachers will be available to help in a variety of ways. While independent study is hard work, it is also tremendously satisfying.

Contact the Independent Learning Centre by mail at: 20 Bay Street, Suite 300, Toronto, ON, M5J 2W1. Web site: http://ilc.edu.gov.on.ca. Fax: 416-314-8575. Phone: 416-325-4388 and 1-800-387-5512.

What It Costs

Currently there is a $33.25 refundable administration fee for each course request. The fee applies to every course offered in the course guide, including full-credit, half-credit, and non-credit courses. The $33.25 fee will be refunded when you have successfully completed the final test and returned certain items. So essentially the course is free, but you are responsible for a few miscellaneous items, which will be itemized in your information package.

Typical Credit Courses by Subject

arts	guidance
business studies	history and contemporary studies
English	international languages
French	mathematics
family studies	personal life management
geography	science

Procedure for Additional Courses

Once ILC has recorded a passing mark for the first unit of your first course, you can request an additional course. The same rule applies for each course request after that. You can request an additional course only after the mark for Unit 1 of your latest course is recorded at ILC and if you have submitted work for each of your other courses within the previous 90 days. More details are contained on ILC's Web site.

QUICK SUMMARY

- Learning is becoming a lifelong process. About one in four adult Canadians participate in some form of education activity every year.

- Universities and colleges all across Canada provide a wide range of educational opportunities for part-time, mature, and evening students.

- Distance learning presents a great opportunity for adult learners.

In this chapter:

- Find out why so many people love their craft or hobby.

- Pick up ideas about a craft or hobby that would appeal to you.

- Find out how others acquired their skills.

- Find out how to do something special for a loved one.

Happiness, at all levels of the workplace, has to do with being engaged.
— Tom Peters, management guru and author

Personal Expression

More than 30,000 years ago, prehistoric man expressed himself by painting images on cave walls of present-day France, Spain, and other parts of the world. Their drawings usually depicted reindeer, horse, bison, and ox. And according to the experts, their paintings were performed with a high degree of skill.

What motivated them to do it? In their quest for an answer to that question, prehistorians have considered possibilities that range from some form of ritual to simple decoration. When the dust settled, it appears that their motive was nothing more complex than creating art for art's sake.

Is it any wonder that 300 centuries later we still derive intense satisfaction and self-fulfillment from the process of creating or making things? It must be in our genes.

Surely you have experienced the feeling of satisfaction and contentment that comes from creating something. Whether it's building a bird house, writing a story, painting a landscape, or making a quilt, as long as you enjoy it, there is more satisfaction in the process of doing than in the final accomplishment. And so it should be. In the book *Are You Happy?* Dr. Theodore Rubin has this to say:

> If you are totally goal-oriented in a success-oriented culture, and if the product is the goal, you have destroyed much of the possibility for happiness in your life, since almost all of your life has to be the process and not the product. If you can't live in peace with the process of living itself, there goes your happiness.

Continuing with that thought, if you enjoy what you are doing and derive considerable satisfaction from the process, you are probably experiencing what we know as happiness. That's a pleasant thought that we sometimes forget.

Have you noticed that as you get closer to completing a project the intensity of your satisfaction increases? A sort of frenzy takes over as you rush towards the finish line. Some people will even postpone eating and sleeping in order to spend more time on their project as it nears completion. Isn't it great that we can acquire happiness from the simple act of doing something as we move through life?

Deep inside we know that creating and doing will bring pleasure, but once we get on the downhill slide to boredom or depression we tend to give up, and it becomes increasingly difficult to take charge of our life and change course. We even forget what to do and where to look for a way out of our predicament.

So what's the solution? This chapter is designed to trigger ideas in your mind that will open new doors and put satisfaction and fulfillment back into your life. There are so many things out there waiting for caring hands to touch it, rearrange it, paint it, or make it. Could those caring hands be yours?

A Bird's-Eye View

What can you do? If, over the years, your life has become a repetition of never-ending boring chores, this chapter will help you get off that treadmill. In this part of the book our aim is to help you find the courage to pursue at least one of the seven options we offer below. Once you get started you will enjoy the sense of accomplishment that comes from creating and doing.

Seven Ways to an Active Mind

1. Try your hand at a craft.
2. Take up a hobby.
3. Attend meetings and events.
4. Join a group.
5. Go places and do things.
6. Create and organize.
7. Do something special for a loved one.

For years, thousands of people have yearned for the time when they would be free from their nine-to-five jobs and able to pursue their dream of spending endless hours at their hobby or special interest. You may be one of them. Whether it's photography, ballroom dancing, or woodworking, this may be the time in your life to resurrect that urge and chase your particular rainbow. If you can't pinpoint exactly what you are searching for, don't be too concerned, for there is a wide range of choices in this chapter that will surely include at least one idea that appeals to you.

Once you make your move and get started in your special pursuit, chances are there will also be surprises in the form of additional benefits. You will make new friends and meet interesting people, visit new places, and expand your areas of interest. You will no longer pace the floor in boredom — you will be too busy enjoying yourself. If you decide in earnest to get involved with one or more of the opportunities presented here it will have a significant impact on your lifestyle.

1. Try Your Hand at a Craft

By far the largest number of options fall under the heading of crafts. The list below is intended only to serve as an idea generator; it is not a comprehensive list of the craft categories. For instance, the list does not include basketry, calligraphy, or needlepoint, which are all very interesting activities. We do not intend to provide a description of the crafts or hobbies, for that is not the purpose of the chapter. If you would like a more detailed list or additional information about a particular craft or hobby, visit your local library or check out one of the Web sites mentioned later on.

If by chance we have referred to your favourite activity as a craft when you think of it as a hobby or a pastime, please bear in mind that the dividing lines are a bit hazy. We have no desire to cross swords with anyone.

A Few Crafts:

Beadwork	Picture framing
Candle making	Pottery and ceramics
Floral design	Quilting
Flower arranging	Sewing
Folk art painting	Stained glass
Hairstyling	Tole painting
Interior decorating	Weaving and spinning
Painting: watercolour & oil	Woodworking and woodcarving

Why Do They Do It?

Crafters have numerous reasons for devoting so much of their time to doing what they love best. Here's what some of them have said about why they do it.

Calming and relaxing:

- *When working on a project I feel totally at ease without a care in the world for I'm mentally immersed in what I am doing.*
- *When I'm painting, I am totally relaxed and able to concentrate.*

A rewarding experience:

- *I surprise myself when I see what I'm capable of doing and that makes me feel good.*
- *I enjoy the finished product, and I like being able to give hand-made pieces to close family members to remember me by.*

An opportunity to be creative:

- *Before I began painting I had no idea that I had talent. Even now, when I look at the finished product I am surprised that I actually made it myself.*

Keeps me busy:

- *I'm not the sort of person who can sit around doing nothing so I might as well do something that I enjoy and be productive at the same time.*
- *I do folk art, and it keeps my mind active. The larger the project, the bigger the challenge.*
- *My husband and I both do crafting. It keeps us busy and we feel it keeps us healthy and happy.*

Gifts for family and friends:

- *I used to spend hours and hours knitting sweaters for all my children and grandchildren. A few years later it was interesting to see the sweaters passed on down the line to the younger kids as they grew into them.*

Mix with other people:

- *I do most of my work at home, but I attend instruction with a group and I enjoy that.*
- *I needed to get out of the house and meet new people. And it affords me time to relax and lose myself for a couple of hours while painting and listening to easy music.*

Make a few dollars:

- *Some people set up shop and sell their crafts in malls, country fairs, craft stores, church sales, and crafters markets. And usually their prices are most reasonable. When I broached the subject of price with one lady she said, "We work for a pittance," and maybe they do.*

For fun:

- *One lady said, "I like doing it, it's fun. Isn't that good enough?"*

Inspiration from an Artist

Continuing with the question of why people do it, here are the reflections of an artist as he speaks of why he paints. Bob Pennycook is an internationally known artist, teacher, and author of instructional books. He usually introduces his books with a brief inspirational message "from the soul." Olga has taken several courses from Bob and she especially likes this introduction from his book *Home for the Holidays*. We hope you like it, too.

by Bob Pennycook

I'm a folk artist for the joy of it. The spirit of the child is still within me and I paint for the pure joy of adding color, texture, and design to almost anything in sight.

But from somewhere inside, I also paint to communicate. And what I want to communicate are steadying forces of life-love, happiness, peacefulness, warmth, and the sometimes hidden beauty in the things that surround us. By using traditional folk art symbols, combined with color, texture, and design, I can paint from the soul and, in the process, still have fun.

For those of you sharing these designs, I hope the spirit of the child in you appears each time you pick up a paint brush and guides you through some new and exciting territories.

And the Winners Are!

Since there are no Canadian statistics available about the extent and health of the crafts and hobby industry in Canada, we have drawn upon some interesting statistics from a survey conducted in the United States. The Hobby Industry Association recently conducted a craft/hobby consumer survey of consumer attitudes and behavior relative to crafts and hobbies. We feel there is value in presenting selected portions of that survey here, because in all likelihood they also reflect Canadian attitudes.

The various needlecraft activities attract the greatest number of participants, with "cross-stitch/embroidery" being the single most popular one. The list below provides a comparison of the most popular crafts reported in the craft/hobby consumer survey.

Participation Rates for Crafts/Hobbies:

Cross-stitch/Embroidery	45 percent
Crocheting	29 percent
Apparel/Fashion sewing	26 percent
Home décor painting	25 percent
Craft sewing	24 percent
Cake decorating/Candy making	22 percent
Needlepoint/Plastic canvas	22 percent
Art/drawing	21 percent

Floral arranging	21 percent
Home décor sewing	21 percent
Scrapbooking/Memory crafts	20 percent

Creations Are Put to Good Use

When Olga was on her sweater-knitting spree a while back, it seemed that I was constantly asking her, "Who is this one for?" Usually she responded by naming a little boy or girl, but one time she said, "This one is for you, my dear." Suddenly I realized that all that knitting really was being put to good use. Nowadays she applies her creative skills to craft painting, producing a variety of attractive pieces. A few of her paintings adorn the walls of our home, but the vast majority of her work ends up as a gift for a friend or relative.

Many crafters would never dream of selling their work, but of course some do. If you are interested in going that route, you may like to take a look at the book *The Complete Idiot's Guide to Making Money with Your Hobby.*

For your information, those who responded to the U.S. craft/hobby survey said this is how their work was used:

Uses for Craft/Hobby Creations

As gifts	71 percent
Home decorations	69 percent
Personal use	62 percent
Holiday decorating	59 percent
Items to sell	16 percent

A Few More Results from the Craft/Hobby Survey

- 80 percent of households surveyed reported that at least one of its members engaged in a craft or hobby.

- The typical hobbyist spends an average of 7.5 hours per week on his or her crafts/hobbies.
- Needlework continues to reign as the most participated category.
- Paper-related activities (rubber-stamping, scrapbooking, and paper crafts) have shown significant increases in participation.
- Bead crafts and candle making show increased participation.
- Crafters experience the benefit of a positive emotional experience.

The Hobby Industry Association also assembled attitudes and opinions of 500 women 55 years of age and older. Here is a summary of what they reported.

- Virtually all mature women (97 percent) have participated in some kind of craft activity in their lifetime.
- Almost 9 in 10 have done some kind of needlework or craft.
- Three-quarters of mature crafters find it relaxing to do crafts.
- Two-thirds like to make things to give as gifts.
- Overall, 6 in 10 women 55 and over can be encouraged to craft more. The best ways to catch the attention of these women and to pique their interest in a craft is through friends and family, magazines, and craft fairs.
- One-third of women 55 and over say they would craft more if they had more time or were retired.

How to Acquire the Skills

How many times have you heard someone say they wish they knew how to do this or make that? If you are one of that group, there is no need to torment yourself any longer. There are many ways to learn how, and a lot of talented people are anxious and willing to teach you. When I wander down the aisles of a crafters marketplace or visit the booths at a one-of-a-kind show I am astonished at the assortment and high quality of work on display. I decided to find out how the crafters learned how to do such beautiful work. I asked a lot of questions and found that they learned from a variety of sources:

- Many crafters learned their skill from another family member or from a friend.
- Crafters learn from magazines, newsletters, books, and catalogues.
- They watch craft/hobby related television shows.
- They attend craft fairs and festivals where they pick up new ideas.
- Craft stores conduct training courses and workshops at their place of business and many novice crafters learn their skills at these courses.
- Many crafters have tried out more than one craft or hobby before deciding to concentrate on the one they like best.
- As with anything else, practice makes perfect.
- The odds are there is a training course being conducted right now in your own neighborhood on the craft or hobby you are interested in. Check your phone book, call city hall, get information from your library, call your local centre for education and training, or contact your local community colleges.

Excerpts from Course Write-Ups

Here are a few actual examples of what you will find when you check out the general interest courses you are interested in. We include these examples to give you an idea of how interesting and informative the courses actually are.

> **Craft in a Night:** Complete a craft each night! This course introduces a variety of craft techniques for creating simple projects. Craft in a Night is a great introduction for the beginner. It is non-intimidating and at the end of each session you walk away with something you created yourself.

Drawing: Along with standard mediums, you learn the white line drawing technique of scratchboard and the art of coloured pencil. Perspective, still life, and portraiture will also be included.

Flower Arranging: Learn to design and create swags, dried flower arrangements, wreaths, topiary trees, fruit crescents in baskets, holiday centerpieces, and more.

Folk Art Painting: Using simple, primitive folk art designs you work on two or three different projects and explore different painting and background techniques.

Quilting: Learn the art of quilting through the introduction of different piecing and appliqué techniques. A small quilted wall hanging or table mat will be made using updated quilting methods.

Stained Glass: Learn to design, cut, assemble, and solder a small traditional stained glass panel.

2. Take Up a Hobby

A Few Hobbies:

Astronomy
Billiards, snooker, pool
Birdwatching
Blacksmithing
Collecting: coins, stamps, etc.
Cooking
Gardening

Interior decorating
Jewelry making
Model railroading
Photography
Weaving
Knitting

Done Any Whittling Recently?

Many of the activities we now think of as hobbies or crafts were at one time carried out by a tradesman or craftsman working 10 or more hours a day to earn a living. The products they made were essential in their everyday lives. When we make the same products today they usually have a decorative purpose. Think of candle making, basketry, and pottery for example. Most people get pleasure from making something with their hands, but in this modern age we have very little opportunity to discover whether or not we have any talent for it. Many talented people go through life unaware of their hidden potential and it lies dormant, never to be discovered.

Next time you're speaking with a 10-year-old boy, ask him if he has done any whittling lately. I wish I could be there to see the expression on his face in response to such a question. Now I ask you, how can a young lad find out what he can do with hands if he has never had a chance to whittle? There was a time when every youngster took pride in his very own pocket knife and the modest carvings he created with it, but now they are denied the privilege of even owning one. Too bad.

Crafts allow you to work with your hands. You begin with an object of little value in itself, then your brain and your hands work in harmony to turn an ordinary piece of canvas, wood, or mixture of clay into something useful and beautiful. It is that process of creating something new that provides the feeling of satisfaction, reward, and even exhilaration. You can stand back, look at it, and say, "I made that!"

The Arm with a Hammer

As a kid in the small southern Saskatchewan town of Lafleche, I often wandered into the blacksmith shop to watch what was going on. As long as I stayed out of the way the blacksmith (can't remember his name) didn't seem to mind. I was fascinated by the intense cherry-red heat emanating from the forge and the constant hammering as the blacksmith pounded a piece of iron into the shape he wanted. For a 12 year old it was magic at work. Every small town had a blacksmith shop, for it was an essential part of the community.

The blacksmith could shape anything made of iron, he could forge-weld, and he could shod a farmer's horse. Now, the horses are at the race track, the small towns have disappeared, and the blacksmiths are producing decorative iron work.

Although the country blacksmith has left the scene, a few dedicated blacksmiths are determined to keep their art alive. It's also a way of keeping the memory of our ancestors alive, and I like that. The Canadian Blacksmith Conference promotes the art of blacksmithing and fellowship among blacksmiths by holding its CanIRON conference every second year. In 1997 CanIRON was held in British Columbia, in 1999 it was held in Calgary, and in 2001 CanIRON was held in North Battleford, Saskatchewan. If I had known about it sooner I may have made the trip to North Battleford, just to stand around and see what was going on. CanIRON's Web site is found at www.geocities.com/caniron.

Excerpts from Course Write-Ups

Once more, here are some excerpts from actual hobby course descriptions. We find them enticing, don't you?

> **Astronomy:** Learn the fundamentals of the solar system, galaxies, black holes, and other heavenly bodies. You will also learn about buying and using a telescope.

> **Birdwatching:** Learn to identify birds by both sight and song. We will focus on migrating hawks, shorebirds, waterfowl, and songbirds.

> **Gourmet Cooking:** Learn to prepare and then enjoy gourmet meals from basic sauces to mouth-watering desserts. You will also learn about traditional recipes from around the world.

Photography: Learn about formal and informal composition, depth of field, natural and fill lighting techniques, use of filters, still life, children and nature photography.

Model Railroading: Learn about track planning, bench work, electrical work, scenery, structures, locomotives, and much more. The course also includes a field trip to a large club layout.

Play the Bagpipes: Apparently, you can learn how to play the bagpipes if you live in the right city. Here's an excerpt from an e-mail I recently received from a friend in P.E.I.:

> *"I retired last Friday and will have more time to devote to things that I like to do. Among other things I have taken up the bagpipes again after a hiatus of 25 years."*

Visit our Web site at www.after50.ca and look under "Resource Links" for a comprehensive list of craft and hobby Web sites.

ACTIVITY # 10:

Please take a moment to complete the chart below.

Crafts and Hobbies	
What's your situation?	
What hobbies or crafts have you been involved with in the past?	
What crafts or hobbies are you interested in now?	
What personal benefits do you hope to achieve?	
When would you like to get started?	

3. Attend Meetings and Events

If you want to know what's happening in your own backyard, pick up a copy of your local newspaper and turn to the community calendar section. There you will find a summary of the meetings and events taking place in your corner of the world. There's no need to be lonely. Get involved, join other folks in your community, and you'll see that there are a lot of things going on. Don't be afraid to take that first step — you will be pleasantly surprised at the friendly welcome you will receive.

Below is an edited list of meetings and events that were advertised in just one issue of a local newspaper. Similar events are going on you your community, so why not give it a try? You may find what you are looking for. If you are hesitant to go it alone, call a friend and break the ice together.

- A chorus group is looking for members.
- A ladies group is holding their weekly "Coffee Break" get together.
- The United Church is hosting its annual multicultural dinner.
- The Bassmasters Club invites fishing enthusiasts to a meeting.
- The Genealogical Society is holding its regular meeting.
- The Historical Society is celebrating its 20th anniversary.
- The library is hosting a workshop for aspiring writers.
- The Newcomers Club invites newcomers to a meeting.
- The Royal Canadian Legion is hosting a breakfast.
- The Scottish Club is holding its annual Burns Supper.
- The Widows and Widowers Club is hosting a dance.

 Go for It!

There are so many ways to keep your mind active. Do crossword puzzles, read good books, start a book club. Play bridge or invite a friend over for tea and plan outings. Don't be afraid to join things on your own if you must; there are always lots of singles. Challenge yourself. Take a trip alone. Meeting new people is wonderfully stimulating.

— Louise Tye

4. Join a Group

Here are a few of the kinds of clubs or groups that welcome new members:

Book review clubs
Camera clubs
Bridge, euchre, and whist clubs
Church groups
Museum and heritage foundations
Drama clubs
Sports clubs: tennis, curling, golf
Garden groups
Horticultural societies
Investment clubs
Service clubs such as Lions and Probus

ACTIVITY # 11:

For future reference, make a note of the meetings, events, or clubs in your community you are interested in.	

5. Go Places and Do Things

When you were working you may have complained about not finding enough hours in the day to get the job done. Now that you are retired you may find yourself with time on your hands. If that ever happens, here are a few interesting things you can do.

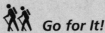 *Go for It!*

Work with your local library to select books to read, and find clubs to join where you can learn, be challenged, and fill a need.
— Stewart McTavish

- Attend a city council meeting.
- Attend a music festival.
- Attend the Senior Games in your area.
- Bake a pie for a neighbour.
- Browse through the library or your favourite bookstore.
- Read a book.
- Do a crossword puzzle.
- Dine out for a change.
- Do some stretching exercises.
- Tidy a closet, then take clothes to Goodwill or the Salvation Army.
- Find your local bingo hall and try it out.

- Go for a bike ride, a walk, or a hike.
- Go to a baseball or hockey game.
- Go to a matinee theatre — the prices are better, too.
- Organize your old photographs.
- Phone or write an old friend you haven't been in touch with for years.
- Take a day trip to the country.
- Take a field trip with your grandchildren.
- Visit a friend in the hospital.
- Visit the art gallery or museum.
- Visit your local courthouse and sit in on a court case.
- Volunteer at your local animal shelter or local school.

Time with Your Grandchildren

You'll enjoy the articles and ideas provided at this Web site: www.mygrandchild.com. It provides a wonderful source of information about that special relationship shared between a grandparent and a grandchild.

Vacation with a Grandchild

Several years ago Elderhostel invited parents or grandparents to bring one or more children aged 10 to 15 on an outdoor adventure. That outing caught my eye so I took my 13-year-old grandson, Josh, for an exciting week of outdoor activities at the Strathcona Park Lodge on Vancouver Island. Josh, now 22, recently mentioned how much he enjoyed that week of rock climbing, canoeing, kayaking, and exploring nature. Give it a try.

ACTIVITY # 12:

Make a note of the places you would like to visit or things you would like to do some day.	

6. Create and Organize

Most of us complain about "the way things are" but never do anything about it. A friend named Judy was annoyed that the retired men at her former place of employment were organized into a club but there was nothing similar for the retired women. Judy got on the phone and in no time at all she created a women's club that meets for lunch once a month. Things don't have to remain undone — if you would like to create or organize something, go ahead and do it. Here are a few examples:

- Organize a group or a club when you see the need.
- Organize a bridge or euchre club.
- Organize a family picnic.
- Organize a family reunion.
- Start up a computer training program for seniors.

ACTIVITY # 13:

What would you like to create or organize?	

7. Do Something Special for a Loved One

Here's an opportunity for you to do something very special for your parents, a relative, or a friend. Send them a "special congratulatory certificate" from the prime minister, the governor general, or the queen. Here's how:

From the Prime Minister

You can arrange for a congratulatory certificate from the prime minister for anyone celebrating a wedding anniversary of 50 years or more or a birthday of 75 years or more.

Submit your request six weeks in advance to: Executive Correspondence Unit, Room 105, Langevin Block, Ottawa, ON, K1A 0A2. Ph.: 613-941-6861.

From the Governor General

You can arrange for a congratulatory message to be sent from the governor general if the recipient is celebrating a birthday of 100 years or more or a wedding anniversary of 60 years or more. There is no need for proof of age or proof of years of marriage. Delivery will take six weeks from the time your request is received. Mail to: The Anniversary Section, Office of the Secretary to the Governor General, Government House, 1 Sussex Drive, Ottawa, ON, K1A 0A1. Ph.: 613-993-2913.

From the Queen

You can obtain a congratulatory message from the queen for anyone celebrating a birthday of 100 years or more, or a wedding anniversary of 60 years or more. To obtain the queen's message on time, you must mail your request along with proof of birth or marriage at least eight weeks prior to the anniversary date.

For proof of birthday you must provide one of the following:

- a photocopy of birth certificate,
- certification of birth by a member of the clergy or notary public, or
- the individual's Old Age Security Number.

For a wedding anniversary one of the following must be provided:

- a photocopy of wedding certificate,
- certification of date of marriage by a priest, minister, rabbi, or Provincial Registrar's Office, or
- an official document or dated newspaper clipping of a previous wedding anniversary.

Mail your request to: Office of the Secretary to the Governor General, Government House, 1 Sussex Drive, Ottawa, ON, K1A 0A1. Ph.: 613-993-2913.

- Thousands of people derive incredible personal satisfaction and enjoyment from working at the craft or hobby of their choice.

- If you are searching for something more, find out what's going on in your community and consider joining a club or group. If you're not a joiner, broaden your areas of interest by attending meetings and events in your area.

- If somebody you love is about to celebrate a significant wedding anniversary or birthday, you can arrange to have a special congratulatory certificate sent from the prime minister, the governor general, or the queen.

"I can only define success for myself, I just don't think it's appropriate or me to try to define a word as important as that for anybody else. For myself, success is, during this earthly pilgrimage, to leave the woodpile higher than I found it."
— Paul Harvey, U.S. news analyst

The Challenge Is Yours

It is our sincere wish that this book has filled a need in your life. We hope that it has caused you to make a start at becoming more physically active. If you are already doing something active, congratulations! That first step is important, for tomorrow it may lead to a truly active lifestyle.

We are equally hopeful that the second part of the book, Active Mind, has triggered an interest that will occupy your time and fascinate your mind for years to come. As a result, we hope that you will never fall victim to boredom, loneliness, or depression.

Now you are faced with the challenge of applying what you have learned and making it work for you. There is a significant body of research to indicate that if you adopt a lifestyle of staying physically and mentally active you will live a healthier and happier life than those who do not. It's up to you to choose the right path.

Mind the Gap

If you have ever travelled on the Toronto subway system you must have noticed the "Mind the Gap" stickers on the doors of every subway car. The full message to passengers is this: "When boarding or exiting the train, mind the gap between the train and the platform." The gap is only about three inches wide, but obviously it presents a hazard for some folks who may trip and fall if not warned. Gaps are something to

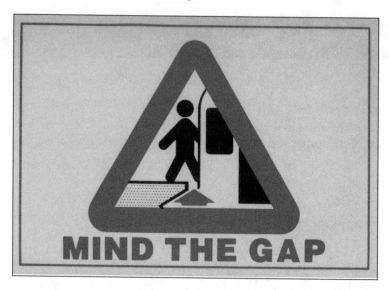

be avoided, and where possible gaps should be reduced or eliminated altogether. A gap is usually the difference between the actual and the ideal situation.

No doubt, there are gaps all around us that we know nothing about, but that's just as well, for we have enough to worry about already. Here are a few personal gaps you may be able to relate to. I'm sure you can think of many more.

- The gap between your actual golf score and what you would like it to be.
- The gap between your actual income and what you would like it to be.
- The gap between the names you can actually remember and those you wish you could remember.
- The gap between how well you feel every morning and how well you would like to feel.
- For men, the gap between how much hair you have on top and how much you wish you had.
- For men and women, the gap between your actual waist size and what you would like it to be.
- The gap between how physically active you are and how active you ought to be.

242

Gaps in Your Life?

For most of us there are gaps in several aspects of our life. What we hope for is seldom actually realized and very few of us are 100 percent satisfied with our situation. In this chapter we will help you concentrate on the gaps that may exist in two areas of your life: what you do for your body, and what you do for your mind.

What You Do for Your Body

This heading does not refer to the pampering you get when you visit your favourite spa. It refers specifically to this question: What are you doing to build and strengthen your muscles; keep your bones strong; help your heart, lungs and circulatory system stay healthy; keep your joints mobile; increase your flexibility; give yourself more energy; maintain a healthy body weight; and yes, even improve your posture?

ACTIVITY # 14:

How's Your Physical Activity Gap?

Answer these next few statements with care for it may be your last chance to give serious thought to what you should be doing to keep your body healthy during the second half of your life.

	Yes	No
• I am satisfied with my present level of physical activity.	❏	❏
• My weight is within the normal range.	❏	❏
• I lead an active lifestyle.	❏	❏

	Yes	No
• I participate in physical activity a minimum of 30 minutes, 4 days a week.	❑	❑

My activities include a balance of:

	Yes	No
• endurance or aerobic activities to help my heart, lungs, and circulatory system stay healthy	❑	❑
• flexibility or stretching activities to help me move easily	❑	❑
• strength activities to help my muscles and bones stay strong	❑	❑

If you answered yes to all the above statements, good luck to you, and we hope you continue on with your active lifestyle.

If you answered no to one or more of the statements, you have a gap that should be narrowed.

ACTIVITY # 15:

Read the first block, then complete the second and third blocks.

1. This is the "Should Be" for an active body

The minimum amount of time spent on moderate physical activity **should be:**

30 minutes of moderate activity 4 days per week.
(The 30 minutes can be accumulated in 10-minute segments.)

2. This is my Actual

In the space below, state how much time you spend on physical activity.

Minutes _____

Days Per Week _____

3. This is my Gap

In the space below, state the GAP between your "should be" and your "actual."

Minutes _____

Days Per Week _____

A Final Reminder: Inactivity Can Hurt
(from "The Healthy Heart Kit" sponsored by Health Canada and others)

Inactive people may develop these problems:

- Heart disease
- Obesity
- Diabetes
- Bad cholesterol
- High blood pressure
- Back problems

- Osteoporosis (weakened bones)
- Cancer of the colon

Activity Can Help
(from "The Healthy Heart Kit" sponsored by Health Canada and others)

Benefits of being active:

Physical Benefits

- Weight control
- Improved cholesterol levels
- Less chance of developing high blood pressure
- Less chance of developing diabetes
- Less chance of developing osteoporosis

Mental Benefits

- Relief from stress
- Increased self-confidence
- Relief from depression
- Better sleep
- More energy — Being active will probably make you feel more energetic. Being active does not take away energy; it gives you more.

ACTIVITY # 16: NARROWING YOUR GAP

In the box below state exactly what you intend to do to narrow the gap between what you are now doing and what you know you should be doing in the area of physical activity. See what you entered in box #3 in Activity 15.

Points to Remember:

- Choose an activity you enjoy.
- Set realistic goals.
- Keep track of your progress in a visible way.
- Find ways to stay motivated. Reward yourself often.
- Don't put if off – start your activity program today.

> **How I am going to narrow my physical activity gap:**

Your statement in the box above may have a profound effect upon your health and well-being for the rest of your life. We wish you well and we hope that as the years go by, you continue to make the right lifestyle choices and enjoy your second half to the fullest.

What You Do for Your Mind

Once you leave the workplace you are cut off from an important network of friends, you are deprived of job status, and your ego suffers. Retirement usually puts an end to many of your relationships. Essentially you have to rebuild your identity, find a new purpose in life, and take advantage of the opportunities available in your retirement environment. In the second part of this book we explored various ways that you could engage in creative, challenging, and enjoyable activities to keep your mind active.

In the Introduction to this book we quoted Charles Kingsley, the British writer who said, "All we need to make us happy is something to be enthusiastic about." And how true that is. The trick is to find that "something" that will get you enthusiastic. But where do you look and how do you start?

It may be that you have already made a good start. Once you become more physically active, the mental benefits will follow just as sure as night follows day. So, the first step is to get physically active, then when the benefits kick in you will have more energy, you will see the world in a different light, and you will have the confidence to tackle many areas of interest that you were afraid to consider just a few short months before.

ACTIVITY # 17:

Read the first block, then complete the second, third, and fourth blocks.

1. This is the "Should Be" for active mind

For an active mind, you should seek out creative and challenging activities that give you a feeling of satisfaction and self-fulfillment.

2. This is my Actual

On a separate sheet of paper, list those activities in your life that positively stimulate and challenge your mind.

Now, list those things you do that are a total waste of your time. Also list people or activities that prevent you from enjoying a more mentally active lifestyle.

3. This is my Gap

In the space below, state the GAP between the "should be" and your "actual."

4. This is how I am going to narrow my Active Mind gap:

It's Never Too Late

The experts say that good health and peace of mind go hand in hand. We believe that, but we also know you have to help the process along with some personal effort. Most good things don't just happen — you make them happen. Here are a few tips to help you find that "something" you can get enthusiastic about.

- Don't put a limit on what you are capable of.
- Surround yourself with people who have a positive outlook on life. Distance yourself from whiners and complainers; they discourage positive thinking.

- Life is not perfect, so do the best you can with the hand you were dealt.
- Visualize what you want to happen and visualize it often.
- Discover what you want and what works for you — not what someone else wants for you.
- Don't put off doing something because of your age — it's never too late. Hazel McCallion, the mayor of the City of Mississauga, is in her 80s, still going strong and showing no signs of slowing down.
- You could live one-third of your life in so-called retirement, so make it a productive, enjoyable part of your life. Recognize that you are not just "passing time."

A Parting Thought

We wrote this book to fill a need. It is enormously important to get the Canadian adult population moving. As you already know, more than half of us are inactive. As stated by Mark Tremblay, a kinesiologist at the University of New Brunswick, we are "pathetically inactive." When our research revealed the magnitude of the problem, we knew we had to complete this book and get it into the hands of every 50-plus Canadian who could benefit from it.

We hope that Get Up and Go will have a positive influence on your life. As a result of reading this book we expect you will take the necessary steps to keep physically fit and mentally active during your second half. It is your life, you are in charge, and you have the power within you to begin living an active lifestyle. You are on the brink of the best years of your life. Go for it. It's easier than you think.

Please visit our Web site, www.after50.ca, where we have listed the Web sites shown in this book and many more, which you will be able to access with just a click of the mouse.

We welcome your comments

If you have any comments, observations, or experiences that you would like to tell us about, we would love to hear from you. Please contact us through our Web site at www.after50.ca, or e-mail us at: jim.olga@after50.ca.